Forthcoming FAST FACTS Books

FAST FACTS to
LOVING YOUR
RESEARCH PROJECT

Brenda Marshall, EdD, APRN, ANEF, is a full professor and director of the College of Science and Health's Center for Research at William Paterson University (WPU) in Wayne, New Jersey. She was the coordinator of the DNP program at WPU (2011–2016) prior to becoming a Fulbright Scholar Specialist in mental health. Dr. Marshall is the author of *Becoming You: An Owner's Manual for Creating Personal Happiness, Fast Facts for Managing Patients With a Psychiatric Disorder* (Springer Publishing Company), and *Fast Facts About Substance Use Disorders* (Springer Publishing Company), and she has published articles and chapters for nursing and psychology textbooks. She has been recognized by multiple organizations for innovative teaching methods in research and was awarded the National Excellence in Research Award (2018) by the American Psychiatric Nurses Association. Her three decades of experience in research and nursing have won her international respect from her colleagues in education, nursing, and psychology.

FAST FACTS to LOVING YOUR RESEARCH PROJECT

A Stress-Free Guide for Novice Researchers in Nursing and Healthcare

Brenda Marshall, EdD, APRN, ANEF

With special contributions from
Tom Heinzen, PhD
Professor, William Paterson University

Katherine Roberts, EdD, MPH, MCHES, CPH
Adjunct Professor, Teachers College,
Columbia University

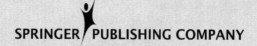

SPRINGER PUBLISHING COMPANY

Springer Publishing Company, LLC
11 West 42nd Street
New York, NY 10036
www.springerpub.com
http://connect.springerpub.com

Acquisitions Editor: Joseph Morita
Compositor: Amnet Systems

ISBN: 978-0-8261-4636-6
ebook ISBN: 978-0-8261-4637-3
Supplementary Appendices to Chapter 15 ISBN: 978-0-8261-5205-3
DOI: 10.1891/9780826146373

20 21 22 / 5 4 3 2

Supplementary appendices for Chapter 15 are available from www.springerpub.com/ffresearch.

The author and the publisher of this Work have made every effort to use sources believed to be reliable to provide information that is accurate and compatible with the standards generally accepted at the time of publication. The author and publisher shall not be liable for any special, consequential, or exemplary damages resulting, in whole or in part, from the readers' use of, or reliance on, the information contained in this book. The publisher has no responsibility for the persistence or accuracy of URLs for external or third-party Internet websites referred to in this publication and does not guarantee that any content on such websites is, or will remain, accurate or appropriate.

Library of Congress Cataloging-in-Publication Data

Names: Marshall, Brenda, 1951– author.
Title: Fast facts to loving your research project : a stress-free guide for novice researchers in nursing and healthcare / Brenda Marshall ; with special contributions from Tom Heinzen and. Katherine Roberts.
Other titles: Fast facts (Springer Publishing Company)
Description: New York : Springer Publishing Company, [2020] | Series: Fast facts | Includes bibliographical references and index. | Summary: "This book teaches the reader not only how to conduct a first research project, but also how to construct an argument, a theory, and critically explore a belief. This Fast Facts book has been written with the novice researcher in mind. It presents an easy guide through the steps needed to be taken when embarking on a research project. It is not a research textbook that intends to cover all aspects of the research study, nor does it teach the reader how to do statistical analysis. For many novice researchers, hiring a statistician, or using the institutional statistician will be needed. This user friendly "pocket support book" can help take the fear out of engaging in research, improve problem solving, and increase the readers interest-dare I say, love?-of research!"—Provided by publisher.
Identifiers: LCCN 2019028552 (print) | ISBN 9780826146366 (paperback) | ISBN 9780826152053 (supplementary appendices to chapter 15) | ISBN 9780826146373 (ebook)
Subjects: MESH: Nursing Research | Health Services Research | Research Design | Nurses Instruction
Classification: LCC RT81.5 (print) | LCC RT81.5 (ebook) | NLM WY 20.5 | DDC 610.73072—dc23
LC record available at https://lccn.loc.gov/2019028552
LC ebook record available at https://lccn.loc.gov/2019028553

Brenda Marshall: https://orcid.org/0000-0001-7500-6990

Printed in the United States of America.

Contents

Part III TEST, ANALYZE, DISCUSS

Contributors

Tom Heinzen, PhD   Professor, William Paterson University, Wayne, New Jersey

Katherine Roberts, EdD, MPH, MCHES, CPH   Adjunct Professor, Teachers College, Columbia University, New York, New York

Preface

Having to engage in a research study—from the staff nurse taking part in a Transforming Care at the Beside (TCAB) project to the DNP student embarking on the DNP project—strikes fear in many hearts. Research, the systematic investigation designed to develop new knowledge, however, is the cornerstone of evidence-based practice and should be a familiar friend of healthcare providers in the 21st century.

Students, nurses, advanced practice registered nurses, administrators, educators, physician assistants, and all other healthcare professionals will be required to:

- Know how to access information related to the best evidence on healthcare provision.
- Work within a framework of standards and constructs that have been demonstrated to be effective.
- Support the research initiatives based in the hospital, agency, or institution.
- Understand the ethical imperative of informed consent and institutional review boards in order to protect the safety and rights of their patients.
- Present findings from TCAB and other research projects at conferences or in publications.
- Make informed healthcare decisions based in the most recently identified best practices.

There are many reasons to love research besides contributing to your education. It is important in our everyday life, empowering a person through improving decision-making skills. The approach presented in this book teaches the reader not only how to conduct a first research project but also how to construct an argument, formulate a theory, and critically explore a belief. This method of conducting research engages the reader in active problem-solving, asking the right questions, finding answers, and being able to understand even the most complex problems. It is through this process a person is able to sit back, look at the data, and determine if the findings are credible. As with most research, the answers usually uncover additional questions that beg for continued inquiry! This is why the last chapter in this book is called "The Beginning: Sharing What Was Learned With the Greater Community."

This book is divided into three sections:

Part I: Define, Clarify, Search, Prepare. This section introduces the reader to the vocabulary of research methods and the importance of defining the problem, identifying the discrepancy, and clarifying the specific problem at hand and the factors that are possible contributors to it. It provides clear strategies for searching the existing literature and refining the aim of the research as well as the question to be studied. For students who are engaging in research for a thesis or DNP project, this first section reflects the first three chapters of the thesis, which develops the proposal. Throughout the book the hourglass of inquiry provides a visualization, identifying where the reader is in the overall research process.

Part II: Starting the Actual Project. This section of the book investigates qualitative and quantitative research designs, methods of data collection, the reliability and validity of data, the sample from the population, and the ethical and legal considerations of engaging in research.

Part III: Test, Analyze, Discuss. The last section of the book is dedicated to the proper collection and analysis of the data (a word that always indicates more than one). It presents the ways that the results can be reviewed, looks at what those results indicate, and discusses how to draw some conclusions from the results. The abstract, which is the last piece of the report to be written, is presented so that the report can be submitted, but that is not the end. The last chapter, The Beginning: Sharing What Was Learned with the Greater Community, introduces the reader to the world of research beyond the paper, including publishing, presenting, and continuing the research by finding funding through grant writing.

Each chapter starts with an introduction and learning objectives. New vocabulary words are introduced with their definitions; tables and "Fast Facts" boxes help to highlight factors of importance, deepening the reader's understanding of the research process. Every chapter also has keywords, references, and links to online websites for those who are interested in learning more.

This *Fast Facts* book has been written with the novice researcher in mind. It presents an easy guide through the steps needed to be taken when embarking on a research project. It is not a research textbook that intends to cover all aspects of the research study, nor does it teach the reader how to do statistical analysis. For many novice researchers, hiring a statistician or using the institutional statistician will be needed. This user-friendly "pocket support book" can help take the fear out of engaging in research, improve problem-solving, and increase the readers' interest—dare I say, love?—of research!

ACKNOWLEDGMENTS

I want to thank my doctoral dissertation chair, Dr. Dennis Mithaug, for igniting the love of inquiry, theorizing, and research in me, a passion that has only grown stronger since graduation. I also want to express gratitude to my mentor, colleague, and friend Dr. Julie Bliss for her interest, support, and collaboration in my research initiatives at William Paterson University (WPU) and for bringing me onboard to coordinate their first doctoral program (DNP). A special thanks to Dr. Tom Heinzen (WPU) and Dr. Katherine Roberts (Teachers College) for their amazing chapter contributions in this book and my students who encouraged me to write this book. Finally, as always, a heartfelt thank-you to my family—Lewis, Olivia, and Megan—for providing me the time and space to write.

I

Define, Clarify,
Search, Prepare

1

Introduction to Research

INTRODUCTION, or *What do you mean, I'm already doing research every day of my life?*

This chapter focuses on examining how we use research in our everyday life. It defines some of the important terms used in research and links them to the things that you are used to doing, like surfing the Internet, for example, and examines the importance of the research outcomes you typically use in a day to support your own health as well as the health of those you take care of.

OBJECTIVES

In this chapter you will learn:

- What we mean by everyday research
- What is an everyday research process
- That it all starts with a discrepancy
- The language of research—same words but different meaning
- The application of the research process to scientific health discoveries

EVERYDAY RESEARCH

What do we mean by everyday research?

Everyday research refers to the thinking processes we engage in and outcomes we experience related to everyday challenges and needs in our normal lives. Ask yourself these two questions:

- How do I know what to believe?
- How can I trust what I know?

We are not always aware of how much everyday research we do because so much of it is habitual. The first time you have to travel to a new place, you might look up where you are going on your phone or put the destination in your car GPS (data gathering). You decide which route to take depending on whether you want to pay tolls, want a scenic route, or want to avoid highways (applying specific criteria). You set your GPS for the destination and go. If the route does not work, you reanalyze the data and revise the plans accordingly. This is a kind of everyday research we do, using our smartphone or smart car, so frequently we do not give it much thought. Other kinds of everyday research might even be more subtle. Here are some examples of how everyday research impacts all aspects of our lives, even when we are not paying attention. Consider the data you had to collect in order to make these decisions that would predict specific outcomes in how your day might turn out:

- What kinds of sounds wake you up in the morning? Phone sounds, music, alarm clock…
- Do you consume milk products, Lactaid milk products, or nonmilk products?
- How do you get to work? Car, mass transit, Uber/Lyft/Via, bike, walk…
- What kind of morning drink do you take? Water, coffee, tea, orange juice…
- How do you choose whom to date? Friends, online dating, hang out in a restaurant/bar…
- How do you decide what kind of toilet paper to use in your home? Plush, soft, strong, thin…

The research we engage in helps us to gather data, test them out, and make predictions of what will happen in the future based upon the results we get. In each of the cases, we have a problem (e.g., get up on time for work) that needs a predictable solution. It might be helpful to consider the research process as a kind of problem-solving approach. The problems listed earlier are so *everyday* in nature that we work on solving them almost subconsciously, but their solutions all follow a patterned process.

THE EVERYDAY RESEARCH PROCESS

Observe a problem
Identify what information (data) you need to make a decision
State the question
Consider what you believe to be the problem and why
Construct the explanation to the problem and solution (hypothesis)
Test the explanation

So now we apply that process to one of the problems: *Toilet paper purchase*

Problem: No toilet paper in the house.
Question: What is the difference between toilet papers?
Data: I need toilet paper; my family likes the idea of the plusher brand.
Nature of decision: I never used anything but my
normal toilet paper, but my
family always asks for the plusher brand. Plush is
more expensive, and I have to
stay within my budget. Maybe if I can find the plush
for less money, it would be okay.
Hypothesis: I have seen all the ads on the plush toilet paper,
and I think that it will not make any difference whether
I use the old kind or the plush as long as they
cost the same amount of money—this way everyone is happy.
Test the hypothesis: Use the plush toilet paper if I find it for less
money; everyone will be happy.

Looking at the scientific method outlined here, we see that the purchase of the toilet paper can easily fit into it. It is important to identify that there is usually a problem that arises, which sets us on the road to data collection, hypothesis development, and trial-and-error behaviors. The research method seems very linear—or step by step—with one leading to the next. In real everyday research, as well as highly specialized scientific research, that process is rarely linear. In fact, consider the name itself; it gives a great clue. It is not called *search*; it is called *research*. Look at something, and then look again and again. Collect the data, run the data, and search them again. Research is not neat. It is not like learning a new dance or practicing how to swing a bat or golf club. It is more like figuring out the perfect way to make a new kind of cookie with multiple ingredients. You have to get your hands into it, figure out what is important, and find out what needs to be included and what should be excluded. It is a kind of amazing game that requires your attention to detail as well as the big picture to get to your outcome, which often is a surprising and unintended destination!

Now back to this toilet paper problem. Take a minute to consider it within the parameters of your own life:

- What is the normal process that you go through to decide what brand of toilet paper to buy?
- What are the factors that influence your choice of toilet paper? You might be swayed by commercials (in other words some good marketing can bias you to one brand or another, without even ever having tried to use it), or you might have your friends or family tell you how good it is (again being biased by the opinions of others).
- What is truly of *value* to you when you are going to buy toilet paper? Is it the cost, the convenience of the place that sells it, the environmental impact factor, the approval of your family/friends, the feel of the paper, or the success of the TV/media advertisers? All these factors are considered variables that impact your decision-making.

Unfortunately, we do not pay that much attention to the process of buying toilet paper or most everything else that we purchase on a regular basis. We are not aware of the impact of others (TV, social media, family, culture) on our own belief systems and our ability to gather pertinent data and then accurately predict outcomes. Value, in everyday purchases and decisions, often falls into impulsive (see it, buy it) or habit (it's what I always buy) decision-making, not the most-predictive-outcome kind of planned decision-making (Marshall, 2009). Impulse and habit decision-making processes do not engage the important process of research of data gathering and evidence-based prediction. They minimize the importance of identifying and isolating factors that can affect outcomes. These two kinds of decision-making (impulse and habit) reflect a kind of faulty research process that uses little forethought, and even less afterthought, until, of course, a problem arises.

THE COST OF FAULTY EVERYDAY RESEARCH

You run out of toilet paper. Your family likes the idea of super plush toilet paper (SPTP), and you see the commercials on TV saying that SPTP really will change your life if you use it daily.

(continued)

THE COST OF FAULTY EVERYDAY RESEARCH (*continued*)

You go to your local supermarket, and you see that SPTP is on sale. In fact, it is offered at a really good price and conveniently placed right next to the check-out counter with a big sign over it: Special Today Only. You grab a 12 pack, buy it, and take it home, replacing the other toilet paper in the house.

Two days later you have a backup in your toilet, which overflows and seeps into the floor, dripping through to the dining room below. You have never had this problem before, and you don't know why it is happening. You call the plumber, who comes and announces that the problem is a large wad of thick toilet paper that is jamming the pipes. The inexpensive, convenient, well-advertised paper has now cost you over $100 in plumbing costs, to say nothing of having to repair and respackle the living room ceiling.

What was lacking here? What kind of additional research before making the purchase could have predicted this outcome and helped you to avert it?

Research: 1: careful or diligent search. 2: studious inquiry or examination; especially: investigation or experimentation aimed at the discovery and interpretation of facts, revision of accepted theories or laws in the light of new facts, or practical application of such new or revised theories or laws. 3: the collecting of information about a particular subject. ("Research," n.d.)

When the inexpensive, thick toilet paper was purchased, the thought (belief or theory) was that it would be something that would be cost-effective in getting its business done, make the family happy, and not causes any problems. As it turned out, that thought (belief or theory) was not correct. The decision to buy the toilet paper was made on a faulty theory, which was influenced by hearsay and advertisement rather than by evidence. The impulse decision-making reflected a response to the environment, not a desire to actually purchase toilet paper that would be effective, make the family happy, and be problem free. This example demonstrates how faulty research can still provide evidence upon which to guide future beliefs and behaviors. Actually, using that toilet paper provided evidence, in the form of a negative (and expensive) outcome, which perhaps caused belief revision, which in turn will change future buying patterns.

APPLYING THE RESEARCH PROCESS

Table 1.1 shows how the research process can be applied to the everyday research example of buying toilet paper.

IT ALL STARTS WITH A DISCREPANCY

Discrepancy: 1: The quality or state of disagreeing or being at variance. 2: an instance of disagreeing or being at variance. ("Discrepany," n.d.)

Everyday research reflects a level of "doing our homework" about the outcomes of our decision-making processes. When we are able to identify the problem, whether it comes to our attention because of an unexpected negative outcome or an unforeseen ethical issue, we are faced with a need for engaging our *problem-solving* skills. Often the problems we face are based upon a discrepancy or a conflict between what exists in our everyday world and the way we think the world is supposed to be. Mithaug (2001) identified that the focus of research

Table 1.1

The Simple Research Process in Everyday Research		
Step	**Description**	**Application**
Step 1	Define the problem; clarify what you want to find out and what you want to have happen.	I need toilet paper; I'd like to get some that my family likes, and I don't want any problems with it.
Step 2	Construct the research question. Collect relevant information and come up with a plan, based on your theory (aka hypothesis).	What is the difference in toilet paper? The ads say it will change my life, my family likes the ads, and my friends say it is soft and plush. I'll go to the supermarket and get the plush toilet paper if it is reasonably priced.
Step 3	Experiment	Use it for 2 weeks.
Step 4	Analyze	Using this brand caused a major plumbing problem that cost me a lot of money to repair.
Step 5	Reach a conclusion	I don't need this plush brand of toilet paper.

centering on human problem-solving skills usually engages in four steps:

1. Identifying a discrepancy between the goal state of a solved problem and the actual state
2. Searching for an operation to reduce that discrepancy
3. Applying that operator to reduce the discrepancy
4. Returning to step 1 to repeat the process until the actual state equaled the goal state (pp. 9–10)

According to this method, the first three steps are repeated until the discrepancy is reduced, or the problem is solved. When talking to researchers, you might find out that the research, though providing some answers, also provided more questions, requiring the researchers to go back to step 1.

Fast Facts

Morbidity, Mortality, and Florence Nightingale

Florence Nightingale worked as a nurse in the Crimean Wars in the mid-1800s. She was moved by the terrible loss of life for the soldiers and was very thoughtful about the discrepancy between what should have been and what was. In fact, for every soldier who died from his battle wound, seven died from infection or disease.

It was difficult to get the right data on morbidity and mortality back then (no mass data collection or data sharing capabilities). Nightingale believed that there should be a way to collect hospital statistics, as well as statistics on disease and mortality, so that future health research could be based on the evidence. This was a second discrepancy that motivated Florence to push forward with healthcare changes. How, after all, can you prove your point when you cannot get reliable, valid data to drive that point home? Her proposal was brought to the Statistical Congress in 1863.

A third discrepancy that she uncovered, often seen as one of the most influential, was that patients should be able to receive treatment from trained nursing professionals so that they could get healthy, but the reality was that those who were delivering nursing care were not trained, but rather "untrained 'pauper' nurses, themselves workhouse inmates" (McDonald, 2001, p. 68).

(continued)

(continued)

McDonald's article identifies how the discrepancy gave rise to the problem identification, which in turn provided the motivation for research and problem-solving. Some other discrepancies that gave rise to changes initiated by Florence Nightingale were:

- What use is science if it cannot be presented in a way that is understandable?
- Why were aboriginal children dying at higher rates than English children of the same age?
- Why were some mothers dying after discharge from normal childbirth?

How might identification of these discrepancies lead to researchable projects?

APPLICATION OF THE RESEARCH PROCESS TO SCIENTIFIC HEALTH DISCOVERIES

The development of vaccines, like the Salk polio vaccine, started back in the late 1800s with the discrepancy that a child who gets sick with a virus should not become paralyzed and die. The first polio epidemic occurred in 1894, and it was in 1905 that research discovered that polio was contagious. In 1908 the poliovirus was identified, setting off investigations into polio immunity. In 1921 Franklin Delano Roosevelt was diagnosed with polio, and over the next three decades, many children were affected by and lost their lives to polio. It was not until the 1950s that the research delivered the first successful vaccine. Along the way research tested many treatments and biological examinations and developed hardware like the iron lung to work at keeping children and others affected by polio safe and healthy. Staying focused on the problem, collecting and analyzing the data, clarifying and stating the hypothesis, testing the hypothesis, and refining the problem led to the eventual development of the vaccine (The College of Physicians of Philadelphia, n.d.).

SAME WORDS BUT DIFFERENT MEANING

In any language there are usually crossover words that look the same but do not have the same meaning. When you hear the word and attach the meaning you knew, it can cause a great break in understanding. For example, in the English language, if you are asked by a British friend about your trainers, he would be asking you about your sneakers, not your fitness pals, and your coach would be your bus, not the person who gives you support on the football field. Another word is *braces*; we would be talking about hardware for the mouth, and the British would be talking about suspenders. It can get even more confusing when you are using an English word in a foreign country where English is not spoken. The words would sound the same but have totally different meaning. Two examples of this that could wind up being a big problem in understanding between nationals are as follows: If you use the word *fart* in Sweden, you might be talking about passing wind, but in Swedish it means speed; accepting a gift in Germany would be a bad idea, because the German word *gift* means poison.

This idea is important when you are beginning to work with research or with researchers. Although we are speaking English, many of the words in research sound like common English words, but they indicate a different meaning. Successfully engaging in research requires that you understand the language. Table 1.2 lists of some of the commonly misused words transferred from everyday English into research. In the following chapters, when a word is used that has a different meaning or nuance in research than its use in common speech, it will be identified in italics and defined. The *probability* of this occurring in each chapter has a *p* factor of <.05.

Probability: p factor of <.05. The author is testing whether or not words that have different meanings in everyday English and research will show up in each chapter randomly or not. A $p < .05$ means the author's hypothesis is that there is a 95% or greater chance that these words are not showing up randomly but because this book is about research and everyday uses. So the author will identify these words because they are not random but, in fact, are included because of their meaning in research.

ROUNDUP

This chapter introduced the process, problem-solving, and language of research. People engage in some level of research every day of their lives, from deciding the most effective method to get up in the morning to determining how to stay healthy by what they eat or how much they exercise. The problem usually presents itself as a discrepancy

Table 1.2

Research Words With Different Meanings in Everyday English

Word	Everyday Meaning	Research Meaning
Anonymity	Secrecy, author unknown. "Authored by Anonymous."	Research condition: No one, including even the researcher, knows the identity of the person (participant) in the study. Specific methods need to be in place to assure anonymity.
Confidentiality	Keeping secret. "Don't worry, I'll keep this offshore account *confidential*."	Only the researcher knows the true identity of the participants in the study. Specific methods need to be in place to assure participant confidentiality.
Reliability	Trustworthiness of a person or thing. "This babysitter is very *reliable*."	How closely a measure (numerical representation of a person, thing, concept…) can demonstrate consistency in results.
Validity	Believable, real. "Not eating more than 1,200 calories a day is a *valid* way to lose weight; believe me, I've done it."	How closely a measure assesses a concept that is being tested by a researcher.
Probability	Likelihood. "If you go to sleep at 9 p.m. you will *probably* wake up refreshed."	A statistical measure that evaluates the chance for an outcome to occur randomly (p factor).
Variable	Something to be considered. "When you buy a car, you should think about whether you want a stick shift; it is a *variable* to seriously consider."	Characteristics that can differ from person to person like sex, gender, age, race, education, and so on.

between what should be happening and what is, in reality, occurring. If what you expect to have happen does not occur, there is a problem. The problem, once identified, needs to be clarified, and the data you require to make a decision need to be collected. Part of this process is to develop a prediction (hypothesis) relating to *if this happens, then* that will happen. Once the discrepancy/problem is clarified, the data are collected, and the hypothesis is established. The hypothesis can be tested and the outcome analyzed. It happens all the time, with almost every decision (big and small) that is made during a routine day. How many decisions did you make today? Can you identify the problems/discrepancies they were associated with, the data you collected, the hypothesis you crafted, and the testing you did? Great, YOU are actively engaging in everyday research!

LINKS TO LEARN MORE

These are some links that can be followed to either learning videos or instructive articles and are found in each chapter before the references.

History of vaccines: History of polio: https://www.historyofvaccines.org/timeline/polio

History of vaccines: The scientific method: https://www.historyofvaccines.org/content/scientific-method

References

The College of Physicians of Philadelphia. (n.d.). *The history of vaccines.* Retrieved from https://www.historyofvaccines.org/timeline/polio

Discrepancy. (n.d.). *Merriam-Webster.com.* Retrieved from https://www.merriam-webster.com/dictionary/discrepancy

Marshall, B. (2009). *Becoming you.* New York, NY: iUniverse Press.

McDonald, L. (2001). Florence Nightingale and the early origins of evidence-based nursing. *Evidence-Based Nursing, 4*(3), 68–69. Retrieved from https://ebn.bmj.com/content/4/3/68

Research. (n.d.). *Merriam-Webster.com.* Retrieved from https://www.merriam-webster.com/dictionary/research

Mithaug, D. (2001). *Learning to theorize: A four-step strategy.* Thousand Oaks, CA: Sage.

2

Finding the BIG PROBLEM

INTRODUCTION, or *From nursery rhymes to the theory of relativity: It's all about research*

Step 1   Define the problem, identifying the discrepancy.
Clarify what you want to find out, what is the discrepancy, and why it is important to you.

Searching for the BIG PROBLEM in the curious case of Jack and Jill. This chapter focuses on learning how to (1) define the problem/identify the discrepancy, (2) single out the BIG PROBLEM, (3) drill down to the present problem, (4) consider the significance of the problem, and (5) develop a researchable question.

OBJECTIVES

In this chapter you will learn:

- A few important definitions
- To find a research problem/discrepancy and make it into a researchable topic
- The importance of problem identification: the case of Jack and Jill
- The need for drilling down and simplifying the problem
- To identify and develop the research question from the problem

IMPORTANT DEFINITIONS

Some of the important vocabulary for this chapter includes the following:

Abstract: An abstract is a brief synopsis of the research study, usually between 200 and 350 words, explaining the problem, the method, the analysis, and the outcome.

Empirical Research: When we speak about something being empirical, we are actually referring to getting information that comes from our observations or experiences in real life.

Observations: When we speak of observations in research, we are not referring to a casual regard that we might pay to a scene or a person, but rather we examine with purpose an event or item of interest. This book will ask you to pay attention to two levels of observations: (1) broad observations and (2) specific data-related observations. Our professional observations of systems, diseases, behaviors, and people can lead us to identify broad topics of interest to research. The focused observations, however, accumulated and recorded under specific conditions after the collection of identified data, create a scientific, verifiable outcome.

Research Problem: If the problem identified by observation is that when one sick person with pneumonia is brought into a ward where surgical patients are recovering, other patients become ill with pneumonia, we have identified a problem, but not yet a research problem. The problem we have identified is too broad for research. In order to engage in researching the problem, we have to narrow down what it is that we want to know. This breaks the research problem down to the following: (1) Is it a problem we want to learn how to describe? (2) Is it a problem we want to quantify in its relationship to other things? or (3) Is it a problem that we want to determine as being the cause of something else? Clarifying what we want to know results in deciding how to go about collecting data.

Design: When we narrow down what we want to know, we need to be able to identify a design to get the facts that will help us focus on the actual data reflective of the question. For example, if the problem is descriptive, the way, or method, to use to gather the relevant information might be surveys, observations, interviews, tests, or frequencies. If we are looking for a relationship, however, we will need to look at two or more aspects of the problem for comparison and examination of relationships between factors. Finally, if we are looking to examine whether one set of occurrences causes another, we would need to actually do an experiment whereby we expose one group to the factor we think is causative, and compare it to another group that is restricted from that factor. The first two designs are considered nonexperimental, and the last one is experimental or quasi-experimental. The choice of design is dependent on what the question is, and it is the most important aspect of the study. The choice of a wrong design will have the researcher collect the wrong data. It is like planning a trip to Florida from Maine and then choosing to compare airfares, when you are interested in going by bus. The facts will not help you get where you want to go.

Hypothesis: A hypothesis is a prediction. It is the if-then statement we learned as children. If I do not do my homework, I will not do well in my studies. In research, we consider what we think might happen or might be the result of our observations or, if we are engaging in an experiment, our experimentation. When a hypothesis is developed, it takes into account those observations we will make relative to the problem we are interested in and the specific research problem we are exploring. The hypothesis must take into account the *variables* that will be affecting or affected by the research.

Variables: Variables are factors that play a role in the event. Variables are very important and will be discussed further in this chapter.

Data: Data are evidence that the researcher can collect and analyze to determine some answers to the research question.

THE PREQUEL

Identifying the discrepancy is essentially the *prequel* step to defining the problem; it is actually identifying and defining *what a problem is* and then singling out one problem to focus on. Something becomes a problem when the prediction of what *will* happen (or *should* happen) is not supported by the actual outcomes. It is often this *discrepancy*, or difference, between what is seen in reality and what is believed should be in existence that motivates a person to learn more about how things work, or why they are not working as they should.

FINDING A RESEARCH PROBLEM/DISCREPANCY AND MAKING IT INTO A RESEARCHABLE TOPIC

It is always interesting to hear people say that they cannot seem to find a topic to research. That is like saying that it is hard to find a pair of shoes or a tie to wear. It is just too broad! There needs to be some guidelines to help choose a topic. For example, if you need to find a pair of shoes, what is the occasion? Do you want to be dancing, running, or just going to work? All these factors (variables) will have an impact on your decision of which pair of shoes is the best for the situation. In research, identifying the discrepancy—like *patients should be safe in a hospital when they take their medications, but some patients are getting the wrong medications*—might help identify your topic (in the preceding case, medication safety). Choosing to focus on one thing you care about, where you work or live, that presents a discrepancy is a good place to start.

Topics for research can be found in everyday life or even in nursery rhymes, advertising, Facebook posts, movies, and TV shows. Here are a few examples:

- *Advertising: Effects of anti-smoking advertising on youth smoking: A review* (Wakefield, Flay, Nichter, & Giovino, 2003): www.ncbi.nlm.nih.gov/pubmed/12857653
- *Social Media:* Eltantawy, N., & Wiest, J. (2011). Social media in the Egyptian revolution: Reconsidering resource mobilization theory. *International Journal of Communication, 5,* 1207–1224. Retrieved from ijoc.org/index.php/ijoc/article/viewFile/1242/597 &a=bi&pagenumber=1&w=100
- *Movies and TV:* Starr, C. R., & Ferguson, G. M. (2012). Sexy dolls, sexy grade-schoolers? Media & maternal influences on young girls' self-sexualization. *Sex Roles, 67*(7–8), 463–476. doi:10.1007/ s11199-012-0183-x

Can you identify the problem and the discrepancy that the researchers might have seen in these three examples? The best way to see if you are right is to follow the link and read the abstract (or synopsis of the research).

Fast Facts

The research we do in the medical sciences usually has to do with things that we have seen or experienced while treating a patient or running a unit, which have not turned out the way we anticipated, or testing to find out if what people hold as a common belief actually is held up with tests in science.

An example of this was demonstrated when, in 1862, Louis Pasteur tested the widely held belief in spontaneous generation, which held that organisms could arise without coming from another similar organism. Using two Petri dishes, one with a sterile agar and one with organisms, he waited and observed for spontaneous generation, which did not occur in the sterile dish. Although his experiments in 1885 were specific to the germs he was testing, the reality he discovered led to breakthroughs in vaccinations against rabies, safer treatment of patients, and reducing the spread of disease. That observation, and Pasteur's decision to observe whether there could be spontaneous generation of germs, answered his question, but it also has had an effect on the way the world looks at germs (Smith, 2012).

If you have taken a hand hygiene course in your studies or if you always think about washing your hands before and after treating a patient, you are using the results of Pasteur's empirical research. What other research could come from a 21st-century problem/discrepancy about a commonly held, but incorrect, belief about handwashing?

THE IMPORTANCE OF PROBLEM IDENTIFICATION: THE CASE OF JACK AND JILL

If we choose now to look at the characters of Jack and Jill from the nursery rhyme as a potential topic for research, here's what we might find. Imagine that the text below is a scenario from a case presented at grand rounds in the make-believe XYZ Medical Center.

THE CONTINUING CASE OF JACK AND JILL: CAN YOU FIND THE PROBLEM?

BACKGROUND: Recently there have been a number of children, boys and girls, coming to the ED at the XYZ Medical Center with head injuries. The latest case (one of 30 cases already treated in the ED) is Jack and Jill. This case follows the same pattern as the others.

(continued)

THE CONTINUING CASE OF JACK AND JILL: CAN YOU FIND THE PROBLEM? (*continued*)

BIG PROBLEM: Head injuries (traumatic brain injuries [TBIs]) in children can cause long-term learning and behavioral problems.

SPECIFIC PROBLEM: An increased number of pediatric cases of TBIs have resulted from carrying water down a hill in the town.

EMPIRICAL RESEARCH: A number of the children have come to the ED after "fetching a pail of water" from a well that was "up a hill." In grand rounds the question was asked about the increased incidence of pediatric TBIs in this ED.

CURRENT CASE STUDY PRESENTED: Jack and Jill: One specific case occurred that brought the medical team together for research. <u>FACTS</u>: *Jack and Jill went up a hill to fetch a pail of water. Jack fell down and broke his crown (fractured skull), and Jill came tumbling after (multiple contusions).*

The team decides to break into three groups: one to *describe* the event, one to examine if there is a *relationship* between this case and others occurring in the neighborhood, and one to investigate what is *causing* the problem. The researchers decide to focus on *age* as a predictive factor (variable) because all of the cases seen in this ED ($n = 30$) involved children under the age of 6.

Descriptive: Age is a factor in the children falling: *Question:* What is the average age of children falling after getting a pail of water from the well at the top of the hill?

Relational: The effect of the TBIs is related to the age of the child falling after getting a pail of water from the well. *Question:* What is the relationship between the age of the children falling and the sustained TBIs?

Causal: Young children fall down the hill because they are too young to be navigating the hill and carrying a pail of water. *Question:* Do children over the age of 6, carrying a pail of water down the hill, fall less frequently than children under the age of 6?

The case of Jack and Jill presented to the researchers related to the larger, global problem of pediatric TBIs and then allowed them to narrow their focus on the variable (age) that they were interested in.

These questions on first look might appear to be good, but there are some important "faulty assumptions." Can you find them?

Importance of Problem/Discrepancy Identification

If you identified four major problems, you are correct!

1. The research problem itself is not clearly defined.
2. There is no stated hypothesis.
3. The actual aims of the studies presented are never identified.
4. The variables of interest are never identified.

We know, from Chapter 1, "Introduction to Research", that the observation of the problem gives rise to the identification of the discrepancy. The problem then directs our attention to considering what data we need to collect and helps us to clarify our hypothesis, which explains the problems and identifies solutions that can be tested. None of those things appear to be present in this case study, so these questions arise: Why do we care to do this study at all? Why is it a topic that needs a research project?

How, in fact, did the researchers decide that age is the important variable? The children arriving after falling are between 3 and 6 years old, but nowhere in the narrative are the ages of Jack and Jill presented, so the determination of the researchers to be focusing on age is questionable. Additionally, the researchers have not given us enough information to make us care about this problem. Why should we be concerned about this problem? In the real world, a lot of research needs to be funded in order to be conducted, and unless the presentation of the Big Problem and the aim of the study are clearly presented, the funding for research might not be found, and the study will not be able to be conducted.

Too often, in a rush to get a research project off the ground and running (all too often the student only has 15 weeks/one semester to clarify the topic), the researcher might identify a vast area of possible interest, then go in a direction that is not identified in the problem. Although a research paper may not require the identification of a discrepancy, the understanding of why this problem has attracted the attention of the researcher is still important and can help guide the study.

Considering research as a method to engage in *evidence-based problem-solving* may help clarify the importance of each of the steps. Research demands the clear identification of a problem. It requires the researcher to actively participate in critical reasoning to identify and explain why things are happening. It mandates the ability to identify what is contributing to the events at hand. Finally, it necessitates that the researcher(s) work at building credible explanations that move the reader toward solving this problem through the identification of risk factors or presentation of logical alternatives or solutions.

The discrepancy is the spark that ignites the research, so it is always a good idea to begin with identifying the discrepancy.

Igniting the Investigation by Singling Out the Discrepancy

The discrepancy, the difference between what is and what should be, needs to be identified. For example, children should be able to be safe when "fetching water," but little children like Jack and Jill are not safe (see Table 2.1). Jack and Jill are two of many children under the age of 6 who have been hurt getting water from a well at the top of the hill. In fact, not only are these children not safe, but they are suffering traumatic brain injuries (TBIs) falling down the hill.

Table 2.1

The Discrepancy in the Case of Jack and Jill

The Way Things Should Be	The Reality We Are Facing
Children in our neighborhood should be safe when they are playing or fetching a pail of water.	Children near the hospital are not safe when they play or fetch water and are winding up in the ED with serious head injuries, that is, broken crowns, concussions, and TBIs.

TBI, traumatic brain injury.

Now it is time to look back at the case at hand. Let's start with what we know; the case of Jack and Jill is one case ($n = 1$), but it is not unique. The ED has seen rising numbers of TBIs from very similar cases over the past 2 years ($n = 30$). How can we rewrite the opening background and problem so that it is more compelling and based in the facts at hand?

Notice how including more specifics, dates of occurrences, number of children affected, ages of the children in this case study, and

THE CONTINUING CASE OF JACK AND JILL: A SECOND, CLOSER LOOK AT THE CASE STUDY

BACKGROUND: Recently, between 2016 and 2019, a number of children, boys ($n = 17$) and girls ($n = 13$) between the ages of 3 and 6 years, have come to the ED with head injuries during the months of November to February. The latest case (one of 32 cases already treated in the ED) is Jack (age 6) and Jill (age 5). This case follows the same pattern as the others: unaccompanied minors playing a game of "fetch the water from the well" sustained serious concussions from falling down the hill when returning to the home base at the foot of the hill.

(continued)

THE CONTINUING CASE OF JACK AND JILL: A SECOND, CLOSER LOOK AT THE CASE STUDY (*continued*)

BIG PROBLEM: Head injuries (traumatic brain injuries [TBIs]) in young children can cause long-term health, learning, and behavioral problems.

DISCREPANCY: Children should be safe when playing or conducting daily tasks, but many children in our neighborhood are being injured just getting a pail of water.

SPECIFIC PROBLEM: There has been an increased number of pediatric cases of TBIs in children between 3 and 6 years of age, resulting from carrying water down a hill in town between the months of November and February.

the ages of all 30 children helps us to better understand the scope and particular aspect of this case.

Importance of Problem Identification

The BIG PROBLEM of TBIs in children is a good place for this researcher to start. Looking at the existing literature about this problem might help the researcher identify some patterns that are similar to the one being experienced in this ED. Considering the discrepancy helps the researcher think about what kinds of solutions are needed. Why is it important for children to be safe during play? What is the big problem that arises if the children are not safe? What factors increase the unsafe situation, and what kinds of solutions might decrease these accidents?

Think of the research process like an hourglass, with the BIG PROBLEM at the top, a problem that covers a broad territory (see Figure 2.1). The problem of TBIs in children is vast and could be a good place to start, especially if the discrepancy is that all children should be safe when fetching a pail of water from the well, but the reality is that children are falling down the hill and suffering head trauma. Identifying and finding literature about TBIs in children will help the researcher make the argument on the importance of finding a solution. The literature can help narrow the researcher's focus to the health risks TBIs in young children present. Left untreated, some children could even die from the results of brain injuries, something that should be preventable. This BIG PROBLEM is the top of the hourglass, identifying the broadest aspect of the problem to be probed.

**JACK AND JILL STUDY—BIG PROBLEM:
TBIs IN CHILDREN**

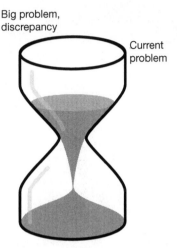

Big problem,
discrepancy

Current
problem

Figure 2.1 Hourglass of inquiry: The BIG PROBLEM and the current problem.
TBI, traumatic brain injury.

DRILLING DOWN AND SIMPLIFYING THE PROBLEM

BIG PROBLEM: TBIs in children cause lifelong problems.
Current Problem: Increased incidence of TBIs in children at a specific hill.
Discrepancy: Children should be safe playing in town,
but they are not; they are getting hurt.

Getting the Facts on TBIs

The problem of children with TBIs, when investigated in the literature, will identify what research has been done in the past, what is
known about TBIs in children, and what is being done to reduce the
number of TBIs. Once the big problem has been defined by the literature, it will be time to narrow the search that is more specific to
the current project. The literature review (introduced in Chapter 3,
"From Hypothesis to Aim/Purpose") will also expose the contributing variables (factors) that have been identified as risk factors for
TBIs in children. This will allow the researcher to focus in on the
case (or cases) at hand, look for any comparative studies, and develop
a specific research question that will reflect the current problem at
hand.

From BIG PROBLEM, the process will move to current problem. It is at this point in the process, therefore, that the researcher has to narrow a bit further. After all, the children in this case are all involved in going up the hill to fetch a pail of water from a well that is located in town. What information, found in published articles or databases, could help narrow the focus, thereby helping the researcher in simplifying the problem?

- Articles about children's falls on hills
- Articles about children who go up hills to get water in pails
- Articles about the difficulty of carrying pails down steep hills
- Articles about the development of muscles required to climb hills
- Articles about the development of muscles for carrying pails down hills

The variables (or factors that are involved in the problem) are numerous, and as you can see, unless you know where you are going, you can get lost in narrowing them down. How many potential factors (variables) do you see in this case study that might contribute to the children's falls? What kinds of questions should the researchers be asking themselves?

- Is the problem with these children falling down the hill local or general?
- What are other variables of interest that could contribute to this fall besides age?
  - Time of year
  - Types of shoes
  - Steepness of the hill
  - Availability of handrails
  - Presence of supervising adults

As you can see, there might be many contributing factors, but these researchers appeared to be interested in the age of the children in this specific case study. One approach to starting this study, therefore, might be to examine statistics that look for similarities existing on falls with TBIs in this age group. This would give rise to the following researchable question:

What is the prevalence (frequency) of TBIs for children under 6 when falling down hills in the United States compared to the prevalence and incidence (new cases) of TBIs for children under 6 falling down hills in our neighborhood?

Examining statistics related to age would allow the researchers to determine if this local problem is actually a *big problem*, or just an unfortunate predicament that is really specific to the children near their ED. In other words, how significant (important) is the knowledge that might be generated by this study? Is the solution they might be able to uncover one that has major impact or local importance? What is the priority of this research? One federal agency that has an emphasis on studying healthcare is the Agency for Healthcare Research and Quality (AHRQ). This agency looks at (and funds) research that can move knowledge from research into actionable implementation of initiatives to improve health and healthcare—research that translates into treatment. "Translational research refers to translating research into practice; ie, ensuring that new treatments and research knowledge actually reach the patients or populations for whom they are intended and are implemented correctly" (Woolf, 2008, p. 11).

Throughout this book, each step leads to another. Identifying the discrepancy leads the researcher to care about a specific event and engage in problem identification, which forms the foundation. From there the researcher drills down to the specifics of the problem at hand, its significance, and the contributing factors. All this leads to the clarification of the research question.

ROUNDUP

This chapter discussed the importance of identifying the discrepancy (difference between what is and what should be), looking into the big problem that is posed by the existence of this discrepancy (i.e., people might get hurt or die), clearly showing how this big problem is related to the problem at hand (project problem/topic), and constructing a question that can be examined to provide some information on the problem and possible solutions.

The Big Problem is the widest aspect of the hourglass, and as you narrow the Big Problem down to your research aim and question, you approach the narrowest part of the hourglass. Any data or information you gather to answer your research question should be specific to *your* aim and related to answering your research question.

LINKS TO LEARN MORE

What is research?: https://www.youtube.com/watch?v=Og4BGyZr_Nk
What is research? The research process: http://www.gavilan.edu/library/LIB99/unit1whatisresearch.html

Agency for Healthcare Research and Quality. Programs and Priorities: https://www.ahrq.gov/programs/index.html and https://www.ahrq.gov/research/index.html

References

Biography.com. (n.d.). *Albert Einstein biography*. Retrieved from https://www.biography.com/people/albert-einstein-9285408

BrainyQuotes. (n.d.). *Einstein quotes*. Retrieved from https://www.brainyquote.com/authors/albert_einstein

Eltantawy, N., & Wiest, J. (2011). Social media in the Egyptian revolution: Reconsidering resource mobilization theory. *International Journal of Communication, 5,* 1207–1224. Retrieved from ijoc.org/index.php/ijoc/article/viewFile/1242/597&a=bi&pagenumber=1&w=100

Empirical. (n.d.). *Merriam-Webster.com*. Retrieved from https://www.merriam-webster.com/dictionary/empirical

Smith, K. A. (2012). Louis Pasteur, the father of immunology? *Frontiers in Immunology, 3,* 68. doi:10.3389/fimmu.2012.00068

Starr, C. R., & Ferguson, G. M. (2012). Sexy dolls, sexy grade-schoolers? Media & maternal influences on young girls' self-sexualization. *Sex Roles, 67*(7–8), 463–476. doi:10.1007/s11199-012-0183-x

Wakefield, M., Flay, B., Nichter, M., & Giovino, G. Effects of anti-smoking advertising on youth smoking: A review. *Journal of Health Communication, 8*(3), 229–247. doi:10.1080/10810730305686

Woolf, S. (2008). The meaning of translational research and why it matters. *Journal of the American Medical Association, 299*(2), 211–213. doi:10.1001/jama.2007.26

3

From Hypothesis to Aim/Purpose

INTRODUCTION, or *Constructing the question and finding relevant data*

Step 2   Construct the research question. Collect relevant information and come up with a plan, based upon your hypothesis/theory.

This chapter focuses on moving from the problem to the development of the research question. Once the discrepancy has been uncovered and the BIG PROBLEM related to the problem at hand, the job of identifying what it is exactly that the researcher wants to know becomes paramount. That question should be tied directly to the reason the researcher has decided to take up this project, defining the aim/purpose of the study. The data that will be collected should be information that provides one or more answers to the research question. Research is undertaken to find some answers, never to prove a theory the researcher has. It is the unpredictable nature of what we might find after analyzing our data that makes research so thrilling.

OBJECTIVES

In this chapter you will learn:

■ How a question requires measurable outcomes
■ The prediction subtext in a hypothesis

- The importance of variable identification
- How to clarify the aim/purpose of your research
- Identifying and avoiding the pitfall of bias
- How to apply these principles to YOUR research project

IMPORTANT DEFINITIONS

Some of the important vocabulary for this chapter includes an introduction to and expansion of the definitions of variables, including independent, dependent, spurious, mitigating, and moderating variables. Variables will be examined more closely in Chapter 5, "The Theoretical Framework." Also, in the same chapter, the types of research, such as descriptive research, relational research, and causal research, will be developed and explored. Finally, this chapter introduces the concept of bias/prejudice and presents the meaning of the null hypothesis.

Variables: Variables in research are measurable factors; they can include the demographics (age, gender, sex, education, income) as well as elements of interest (e.g., drinking patterns, nursery rhymes, study habits). The word *variable* in English usually indicates something that is changeable. In research, variables can be constant (e.g., sex), changeable (e.g., weight, height), an agent of change (e.g., exercise hours), or something that has been altered (e.g., health status). Variables will be discussed in more depth in Chapter 5, "The Theoretical Framework."

Independent Variable: The independent variable is the factor that can be manipulated or changed.

Dependent Variable: The dependent variable is the factor that is acted upon or changed.

Spurious Relationship: In a spurious relationship an element in the research *appears* to have some causal relationship with the dependent variable but is actually not related at all. The variable might just be coincidental, or it may be a variable that is affected by another factor, a third variable, which has not been identified.

Mitigating Variable: This factor can affect both the independent and dependent variables but is not being identified as either. This is sometimes called a confounding variable.

Moderating Variable: This factor, unlike the mitigating variable, can affect the strength of a relationship between independent and dependent variables.

Descriptive Research: This kind of research frequently uses surveys to get information that can describe an event or situation. It presents information on a group, phenomenon, or problem.

Correlational Research: This research identifies relationships between variables.

Causal Research: Causal research investigates whether the independent variable is the factor causing a change in the dependent variable.

Bias/Prejudice: Bias or prejudice in research is not unlike bias/prejudice in life. It refers to having a personal belief (negative or positive) that alters the person's ability to render a nonjudgmental evaluation.

Null Hypothesis: The null hypothesis is actually what the researcher is attempting to disprove. For example, if my hypothesis is that Zoe wears shoes a size too small, then the null hypothesis would be that Zoe does not wear shoes a size too small.

WHAT IS A RESEARCH QUESTION?

A better way to frame this is to ask, What is a researchable question? How do normal questions differ from the research question? During the course of any given day, many questions are asked and answered; not all of them are researchable questions. In Chapter 2, "Finding the BIG PROBLEM," three specific kinds of questions were identified: one that examined facts that described an event, one that looked for relationships between factors in the event, and one that looked for causation. The research question will identify the variables of importance and guide the researcher in the act of gathering and analyzing data. It serves to refine the problem and direct the research.

Constructing a Researchable Question

Let's look back at the case of Jack and Jill from Chapter 2, "Finding the BIG PROBLEM." The researcher has (1) identified the Big Problem—health impact of traumatic brain injuries (TBIs) on children; (2) narrowed the problem to the local event—increased TBIs in children between 3 and 6 years old after falling down a hill; and (3) identified the hypothesis—perhaps the age of the children is a contributing factor to the increase in TBIs. As was discussed in Chapter 2, "Finding the BIG PROBLEM," there were many possible variables that the researchers could have looked into to construct their question, but they chose age. When you are looking at your own project, you will also be facing the need to narrow your focus to one or two factors to research; sometimes this works out the first time, but more often than not, researchers review the factors surrounding the problem multiple times before coming up with a final researchable question.

THE CONTINUING CASE OF JACK AND JILL: CONSTRUCTING A RESEARCHABLE QUESTION

BACKGROUND: Recently, between 2016 and 2019, there have been a number of children, boys ($n = 18$) and girls ($n = 14$), between the ages of 3 and 12 years, coming to the ED with head injuries during the months of November to February. The latest case (one of 30 cases already treated in the ED) is Jack (age 6) and Jill (age 5). This case follows the same pattern as the others: unaccompanied minors playing a game of "fetch the water from the well" sustaining serious concussions falling down the hill when returning to the home base at the foot of the hill.

BIG PROBLEM: Head injuries (traumatic brain injuries [TBIs]) in children can cause long-term health, learning, and behavioral problems.

DISCREPANCY: Children should be safe when playing or conducting daily tasks, but many children in our neighborhood are being injured just getting a pail of water.

SPECIFIC PROBLEM: Increased number of pediatric cases of TBIs in children between 3 and 6 years old resulting from carrying water down a hill in the town.

The discrepancy identified was that children should be safe when playing on the hill, but they are not. What are all the variables that make playing on this hill unsafe for children? There are a number of ways to look at this problem.

- If we are looking to find a practical reason for the falling and therefore a good solution to it, we would need to collect specific data. Our researchable question could be "Why are the children falling down the hill?" or "What are the risk factors that make playing on the hill dangerous?"
- If, on the other hand, we are looking at preventing TBIs in young children playing the "fetch a pail of water" game at the well on the

hill, the researchable question would be "How can head injuries be prevented when children are playing on the hill?"

Clearly, before a researchable question can be constructed, the reason (aim/purpose) for engaging in this research needs to be clarified.

PREDICTION AND HYPOTHESIS

Let's look at three distinctly different hypotheses (predictions) on this same problem of why children are falling and sustaining TBIs when playing the fetch-a-pail-of-water game:

- **Age:** Age is the determining factor in the risk of falls that result in TBIs. Children under the age of 6 are at a higher risk of falling and sustaining a TBI than older children.
- **Risk-Taking Normalization:** These accidents are eerily reflective of childhood nursery rhymes, which normalize the action of risk-taking by children (e.g., "Jack and Jill," "Humpty Dumpty," "Little Red Riding Hood").
- **Winter Seasonal Weather:** All of the 30 cases seen in XYZ Medical Center occurred between November and February. These months are colder than the others and frequently have snow, ice, and rain that covers the ground, making it difficult to walk, run, or play fetch a pail of water.

For each of these hypotheses, let's consider what kind of data would need to be collected to establish the credibility (believability) of the hypothesis.

Each one of these hypotheses may have multiple different questions, and the researcher should investigate the multiple ways of asking the questions, because the data collection will depend on what the question focuses on. One question for determining whether the child's age is a factor in the falls with TBIs could be: *Does a child's age of less than 6 years increase the risk of a TBI with falling down the hill while "fetching a pail of water"?*

What are the variables of interest? They are the child's age and engaging in fetching a pail of water. Data that could support this answer might include:

- A chart review of all TBIs in the past 5 years coming to the XYZ Medical Center, looking specifically at the age of the child and the situation resulting in TBIs (i.e., were they playing fetch a pail of water at the well?)

- A review of previous studies identifying children playing games on hillsides (like fetch a pail of water) that resulted in TBIs, examining the ages of the children who got hurt
  - Are there any other ways you can think of getting information on the age of children sustaining TBIs while falling down hills?

The second hypothesis identified different variables and would require a different method for answering the question—variables of interest: knowledge of nursery rhymes, normalization of risk-taking, age. The research question might be: ***Does knowledge of nursery rhymes increase the normalization of risk-taking in young children?*** How can this information be gathered?

- Look for evidence to support that risk-taking can be normalized by exposure through literature.
- Identify how many nursery rhymes include risk-taking without any serious health outcomes to children.
  - What are some other ways that you might find support for this hypothesis?
  - Whom would you be interested in interviewing/surveying for this?

The third hypothesis identified the *winter season* as a possible factor in the events. The variables of interest might include age of children, number of seasonal falls, and falls during specific winter months for children playing fetch a pail of water. This could give rise to the researchable question of "***Do children playing fetch a pail of water on the hill have a higher incidence of TBIs during the winter season than those in the summer season?***" or "***What is the prevalence of pediatric ED visits related to TBIs from falling down hills during winter months compared to other seasonal months?***"

Some possible data collections for investigating this hypothesis could include:

- A 5-year chart review of pediatric TBIs from the hill, separating the seasons in which those TBIs occurred
- A 5-year chart review of all pediatric TBIs, examining the seasons that they occurred in
- A review of weather patterns over 5 years, comparing wintry mix (snow, sleet, freezing rain) and subsequent ED visits with TBIs
  - Can you identify other ways to find some background support for investigating seasonal impact on TBIs?

Fast Facts

Getting Overwhelmed

Starting out on a research project is exciting, and just like anything else that is new and exciting, sometimes all the choices can become overwhelming. Consider buying a car, for example. First you decide that you want to buy a car.

SO you make the first decision: I'll buy a car. Then you need to decide what car to buy. This decision might depend on many factors: how expensive the car is, where you live, whether to buy a used or new car, what kind of car you want, features in the car you need.

SO you shop online. The choices are overwhelming, and you are inundated with requests from car dealers all over the nation. You can give up or try another way.

SO you go to a local car dealer. There you are faced with many decisions: Which make, model, year, and color should you choose? What kinds of accessories do you want? Should you lease or buy? How many miles do you travel a year? Still overwhelming. You can give up or try another way.

SO you call a trusted friend, who starts asking all the first-line questions again, but this time you are able to focus on what is really important for you. You take a few breaths and consider what is most important. What are your resources? What do you want from this car: speed, dependability, size, color, something else?

The research process is like buying that car. It helps to know why you are doing it (besides graduating from a program). It also helps to have some parameters, like how much time you have to spend on it and how easily the data you need will be accessible to you. You will have to spend a lot of time answering the same questions again and again. Know what you are looking for and where you can find the information.

Remember: You may want to buy an expensive sports car, but if you only have the money for a mini sedan, then reframe what you need to have in that car. The clearer you are when asking the research question, respecting the parameters you need to work in, the less overwhelming the process will be.

IMPORTANCE OF VARIABLE IDENTIFICATION

If my research question is "What is the mean blood pressure (BP) of women at a community college between the ages of 19 and 26?" all I want to know is the average BP of women between the ages of 19 and 26 in that specific school, so the only variable I need to collect would be BPs from women between the ages of 19 and 26 at that school.

If, instead of the average BP of women, my research question is "Is there any difference between the average BP of women between the ages of 19 and 26 at XY school and men between the same ages?" then the only data I need would be BPs from men and women at XY school between the ages of 19 and 26.

Once you have identified your research question, the variables that need to be investigated should be clear. Your researchable variables will be what will drive your research study. When you follow the process of big problem (discrepancy), specific problem, question, variables, refining question, and identifying aim/purpose, you will find the road map to your research study opening up before you. When you identify the purpose of your research, you will be looking back into the discrepancy and how it gave rise to your question.

CLARIFYING THE AIM/PURPOSE

It is at this stage that the researcher needs to be refocusing on the purpose of this study and the development of the specific research question that will be answerable by the data collected. As we discovered earlier in this chapter, each problem has multiple possible researchable questions and projects associated with it. Part of the process will be to refine the researchable question and focus on the data that will help you to reach some answers.

For simplicity sake, let's hold onto the Jack and Jill case study. The discrepancy was that children were getting hurt playing fetch a pail of water on a nearby hill. The researcher needs to identify what kind of solution this research might be able to discover: Is it one that relates to playtime safety? Zoning? Policy regarding parental supervision? Accessibility of the hill during winter months by unsupervised children? Or is it just raising awareness of the danger?

The question for the researcher is, Why undertake this project? What does the researcher hope to accomplish?

What the research should be able to do is solve the identified aspect of the problem of young children getting TBIs when playing *that* game on *that* hill. The three stated hypotheses include the age of the child, nursery rhymes as normalizing risk-taking, and the impact of weather on accidents resulting in TBIs. For this exercise, we will take the first hypothesis regarding age. So, What do we know about young children and head injuries? How can head injuries during other sports/games be avoided? Is there a way to protect the young children when they play?

To construct the argument around this hypothesis, (1) state the facts, (2) lead the reader to the discrepancy, and (3) state the hypothesis supported by the facts.

THE CONTINUING CASE OF JACK AND JILL: CONSTRUCTING THE ARGUMENT AROUND A HYPOTHESIS

1. Fact: All children should be safe when playing a game of fetch a pail of water.
2. Fact: Children in other sports who can sustain injuries due to falling (i.e., bike riding, skiing, some contact sports) protect their heads from injury by wearing helmets.
3. Fact: Helmets have been demonstrated to be effective mechanisms to reduce TBIs in kids once the sport has been identified as high risk for TBIs.

But

Deduction: Many children and parents are not even aware that they are not safe when playing fetch of pail of water on the hill, so they do not know to take precautionary measures.

Hypothesis: Young children playing fetch a pail of water on XY hill are at high risk of TBIs from falling down the hill and breaking their crowns. **THEREFORE:** The *purpose* of this study will be to raise the level of awareness of parents to the risk of young children playing fetch a pail of water without proper headgear.

Possible Research Questions Arising From the Facts and the Hypothesis

- What is the level of awareness of parents concerning the risk of TBIs in young children from playing *fetch a pail of water*?
- What is the relationship between parents' knowledge of the risk of TBIs in young children playing *fetch a pail of water* and their willingness to have their child wear protective headgear during the game?

- Does the wearing of headgear by children under 6 years of age during *fetch a pail of water* have any impact on the number of TBIs?

Identifying the Aim of the Research and Narrowing the Variables

Choose any of the three preceding research questions to determine the aim of the research. Compare your answers with those in Table 3.1. Remember, there can be more than one way to look at a problem and more than one question to be asked, and the variables of interest will arise from the question and the aim of the study.

The *aim/purpose* of the research will be driven by the research question, which is guided by the discrepancy and hypothesis to problem-solve.

The *study question* includes in it the aim/purpose and the variables.

So the *BIG PROBLEM* has not changed; it is still TBIs in children, and the narrowed focus of the current Jack and Jill study will be one of the three questions listed earlier.

The general *hypothesis* that is supporting these three directions of study is that knowledge, awareness, and attitudes toward protective headgear during *fetch a pail of water* can have an impact on decreasing TBIs in children near XYZ Medical Center.

As the researcher narrows the variables of interest down, the process goes toward the narrow aspect of the hourglass.

Table 3.1

Questions, Aims/Purposes, and Variables of Interest for the Continuing Case of Jack and Jill

Question	Aim/Purpose	Variables of Interest
Research question 1	Assess awareness of risk by parents	Knowledge Level of awareness of risk for TBIs
Research question 2	Assess knowledge and intentional behaviors	Knowledge of TBI risk Attitude toward protective headgear Behavior
Research question 3	Assess impact of using headgear on incidence of TBIs	Use of headgear Incidence of TBIs

TBI, traumatic brain injury.

THE BIG PROBLEM: IMPACT OF CONCUSSION/TBIs IN CHILDREN

Focused problem: Lack of parental awareness of prevention with headgear increasing the ***prevalence*** *of TBIs*

Question: What is the parental level of awareness of risk of TBIs in young children from playing *fetch a pail of water*?

BELIEFS AND HYPOTHESIS

Time to explore and clarify your own beliefs about what will be learned (the hypothesis). Sometimes people want to conduct research to prove that they are correct in their thinking. This kind of approach can undermine the study by automatically introducing bias to the process. Another good word to associate with bias, when you are doing research, is *prejudice*. If you are starting your research already prejudiced toward a specific outcome, you might not be able to see how you are manipulating the actual research toward the end you want. When this happens, the whole study becomes tainted and unusable.

The difference between a study free of bias and one that is biased can usually be determined by looking at the hypothesis and the aim of the study. Table 3.2 presents two studies on the same topic: TBIs in children fetching a pail of water. These studies, however, look at the impact of nursery rhymes on a child's probability of taking risk (risk-taking normalization). There is one study with inherent bias and one without. Can you see the difference?

Table 3.2

Problems, Hypotheses, and Aims for the Continuing Case of Jack and Jill		
Big Problem	**Hypothesis**	**Aim/Purpose**
TBIs in young children	Common nursery rhymes impact social norms and increase a child's likelihood of taking risks that can result in TBIs.	To compare the prevalence of TBI-causing behaviors in children's nursery rhymes with the national prevalence of TBIs during playtime for young children (under 6).

(continued)

Table 3.2

Problems, Hypotheses, and Aims for the Continuing Case of Jack and Jill (*continued*)

Big Problem	Hypothesis	Aim/Purpose
TBIs in young children	Common nursery rhymes (like "Jack and Jill") impact social norms and increase a child's likelihood of taking risks that can result in TBIs.	To prove that children who are familiar with nursery rhymes like "Jack and Jill" are more likely to suffer TBIs before they are 6 years old than children who are not familiar with the "Jack and Jill" nursery rhyme.

TBI, traumatic brain injury.

Examining the Two Studies

Study 1

This project is going to look into the prevalence of risk-taking behaviors and injuries in the nursery rhymes and compare them with the national prevalence of TBIs in children under 6 years of age. The researcher does not know what will be discovered, whether there is any correlation (relationship) between these two numbers, or whether the children with TBIs are even familiar with nursery rhymes. The first researcher is simply looking for a possible relationship between these two occurrences.

So what exactly would the researcher be able to discover based upon the questions? This kind of research would allow the researcher to report (1) the prevalence of injury in nursery rhymes and (2) establish whether there is a relationship between the occurrences. In either case, showing a relationship between childhood injury and prevalence of risk-taking in nursery rhymes would not establish any cause. It would, however, start a dialogue that could result in another study looking specifically at those rhymes resulting in injury and parents' attitudes toward independent risky play for children. **Correlation (relationship) between two factors (variables) does not indicate any causation.** Just because two things happen at the same time does not mean that one has caused the other. This is important to remember as you progress through the research process.

Study 2

If you identified study 2 as the one with inherent bias, you are correct! The aim of this study was to **prove** the hypothesis, not to investigate if it had merit. By determining that the research will prove a point, the researcher might *cherry-pick* the subjects or only pick the ones that agree with him or her and present an argument that does not take into consideration the alternate hypothesis (also known as the null hypothesis), which would state that children who read nursery rhymes are less likely to have TBIs than those who do not.

EINSTEIN ON RESEARCH

Albert Einstein had some beliefs that were contrary to the quotidian thoughts of the day. One of those ideas was that rather than thinking of the universe in a constant state of instability, he thought that it was fixed in time and space. In conducting his research, Einstein discovered that the universe was indeed in flux, and working alongside Edwin Hubble the astronomer, he was able to determine that the universe was expanding.

Einstein's love of research is demonstrated by his belief that research is a kind of play, and that in order for us to come to logical conclusions, we play with our ideas to see where they take us. (Biography.com, n.d.; Scarfe, 1962)

**If we knew what it was we were doing,
it would not be called research, would it?
—Albert Einstein (Stedman & Beckley, 2007)**

Novice researchers, and even some with plenty of experience, can be enticed by the thought of proving to others what they personally hold to be a true fact. Research we can count on depends on the impartiality of the researcher to examine the facts as they appear, not as we want them to appear. Especially in research that has so many lives and health depending on it, bias/prejudice should not interfere with outcomes.

LOOKING AT *YOUR* RESEARCH PROJECT

Take a minute now to consider your own research project.

- DISCREPANCY: What have you decided is the discrepancy that is worth investigating?
- BIG PROBLEM: Do you have a BIG PROBLEM identified? How is the Big Problem related to the problem at hand? Is the BIG PROBLEM clear?

- NARROWED/FOCUSED PROBLEM: Can you learn about that BIG PROBLEM by looking at previous research? Can you explain how this BIG PROBLEM is related to your project/study's topic?

- AIM/PURPOSE: Have you been able to drill down and identify why you are doing this research (aside from the fact that you have been told you have to do it to graduate/get paid/get a passing grade)? Is the purpose of your study without prejudice/bias? Are you trying to prove something or investigate a situation?

- RESEARCH QUESTION: Finally, what exactly is your research question? It should be a direct reflection of the aim/purpose of the study. Your research question should have clarity so that anyone looking at the question will be able to see what variables you are investigating.

ROUNDUP

This chapter discussed the importance of identifying the discrepancy (difference between what is and what should be), looking into the BIG PROBLEM that is posed by the existence of this discrepancy (i.e., people might get hurt or die), clearly showing how this big problem is related to the problem at hand (project problem/topic), clarifying the researcher's belief about how this discrepancy might be related to the problem (hypothesis), and developing an aim/purpose to the study to find some answers to the research question.

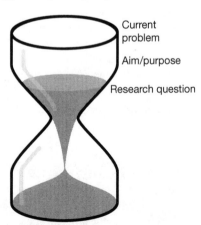

Figure 3.1 Hourglass of inquiry: The aim/purpose and the research question.

The Big Problem is the widest aspect of the hourglass, and as you narrow the Big Problem down to your research aim and question, you approach the narrowest part of the hourglass (see Figure 3.1). Any data or information you gather to answer your research question should be specific to *your* aim and related to answering your research question.

LINKS TO LEARN MORE

What is research? https://www.youtube.com/watch?v=Og4BGyZr_Nk
What is research? The research process http://www.gavilan.edu/library/LIB99/unit1whatisresearch.html

References

Biography.com. (n.d.). *Albert Einstein biography.* Retrieved from https://www.biography.com/people/albert-einstein-9285408

Scarfe, N. V. (1962). Play is education. *Childhood Education, 39*(3), 117–120. doi:10.1080/00094056.1962.10726996

Stedman, R., & Beckley, T. (2007). I we knew what it was we were doing, it would not be called research, would it? *Society & Natural Resources, 20,* 939–943.

4

Why We Review the Literature

INTRODUCTION, or *Why review the literature?*

This chapter discusses the importance of the review of the literature on the development of the research project and the supporting facts for your hypothesis. It's good to think of the review as a kind of exploration. It will be the time when you delve into your BIG PROBLEM and specific problem topics to refine and clarify your research project. This chapter also presents ways to identify where to look for articles, which articles are pertinent, and methods for reading and synopsizing articles. Finally, it demonstrates how this step in the process helps the researcher refine the research question, narrow down the variables of interest, and identify a design for the project.

OBJECTIVES

In this chapter you will learn about:

- The importance of the literature review: time for exploration!
- How extensive a literature review should be
- Avoiding the mousetraps and refocusing if you fall into one!
- Benefits from the literature research experience
- Where to start and how to refine: after the aim and research questions come variables, keywords, and databases

- Getting organized:
    - Using tables and charts for organizational purposes
    - Writing a brief review of articles
- Finding the gaps in the existing literature

IMPORTANT DEFINITIONS

Some of the important vocabulary for this chapter includes the following:

Literature Review: An examination of recent and seminal articles about a specific topic, group, or theory will be determined by the reason you are doing it. If you are looking to support changing a method of patient care to a more up-to-date, evidence-based way, only a brief review of a few articles might be required. If, on the other hand, you are looking to conduct research for a master's thesis, DNP project, or doctoral dissertation, the review should be more extensive and comprehensive. The articles should be both relevant and recent, except when your review is establishing a timeline, which would then include any article reflective of the times of interest.

Seminal Articles: Seminal articles are also called landmark articles. Sometimes it is important to review the first-published articles that established the importance of an idea, theory, or discovery. Despite the year of publication, which might be older than 10 years, it is often supportive and informational to include a seminal article on the topic.

Variables (again): Variables in research are measurable factors; they can include the demographics (age, gender, sex, education, income) as well as elements of interest (e.g., drinking patterns, nursery rhymes, study habits). The word *variable* in English usually indicates something that is changeable. In research, variables can be constant (e.g., sex), changeable (e.g., weight, height), an agent of change (e.g., exercise hours), or something that has been altered (e.g., health status).

Keywords: Keywords are of great importance when searching a topic. The more focused the keywords, the more focused your search of the literature will be. If you are searching alcohol consumption on college campuses and you put "Alcohol consumption" in Google, you might get over 1,240,000,000 results. By adding "college campuses" to the search, you might reduce it to 548,000,000. Add "freshmen" to the search terms, and it increases to 665,000,000. As you add more adjectives, focusing on what you want to know, the results should get smaller and smaller.

Gaps in Literature: As you collect your literature and evaluate what has been reported on in the past as well as the current evidence on your topic, you will be looking for any gaps. Examining the recently published literature reviews on your topic can be a good way to determine the level of existing knowledge and also help to identify where more information is needed. The area that needs more information is the "gap" in the literature.

Databases: Online databases simplify the search for articles, as long as you know what you are looking for and which database would be the best to use to find your articles. For example, Google Scholar (www.scholar.google.com) is a search engine that crosses disciplines to identify scholarly literature on different topics. PsyArticles (http://psyarticles.com) only examines the web for articles related to psychology. Once you have determined your research topic, it is important to decide which database will give you the most relevant articles. You can use more than one database. If a librarian is available when you are conducting your research, the librarian can assist you in focusing your search in specific databases at your institutions.

THE IMPORTANCE OF REVIEWING THE LITERATURE

You have entered the first realm of exploration as you take off into the literature review. Knowing what happened before (by reading what has been published) can help make more informed decisions on how to proceed in the future. Taking the topics from Chapters 1, "Introduction to Research," and 2, "Finding the BIG PROBLEM," imagine if you knew that the toilet paper you were about to buy was no good for people with septic tanks or that children who go up the hill to fetch pails of water without a helmet on might come tumbling down and get a head injury! Reviewing what has been written on a topic helps to formulate a clearer understanding of the situation, identifies common variables between topics, and highlights what is already known by people working in the specific field that is under scrutiny. Once we get a handle on the existing knowledge about a topic, we are able to see where (and sometimes "if") the project at hand adds to the known literature.

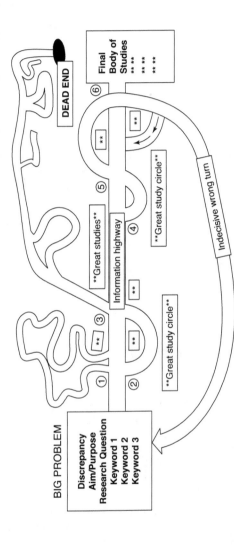

Figure 4.1 Map to a successful literature review. Follow the map from the BIG PROBLEM to reviewing the final body of works found on the informational highway.

** Good studies (usually able to be seen close to the highway; may occur in clumps, in the form of references from other studies).

Exit 1: One way, interesting, but nonproductive side trip. Time-consuming, but you can get back onto the highway.

Exit 2: Great study circle; never lose sight of the highway.

Exit 3: Appealing, maybe even exciting on some turns, but ends up in a dead end. Big waste of time.

Exit 4: Great study circle; never lose sight of the highway.

Exit 5: Indecisive wrong turn onto a bridge in the wrong direction. Be sure to take the jug handle back to the highway, or you will end up where you started and unsure about the value of your topic and research question.

Exit 6: The final goal, a place to sit and review all the studies you have collected on your trip!

The literature review is like an unfolding map that can take you from *what you want to know* along a highway of *what is already known* to your destination of why what you will be doing is important to help provide more understanding to what will be known (see Figure 4.1). It is an exciting journey and can sometimes seem overwhelming, but having a good idea of where you are going will help make getting to your destination less scary!

COMMON QUESTIONS AND MOUSETRAPS

How Extensive Should My Review of the Literature Be?

It is important to know why you are interested in doing this research when considering how deep to look into the existing literature.

WHY AM I DOING A LITERATURE SEARCH?

If you are reading this book, it is assumed that you are embarking on the kind of project that will include some research. There are different levels of projects, from the *I just want to know the project* to the *I want to engage in a meaningful research study and publish my findings*. Knowing why you are doing this study will help you determine how in-depth your literature search should be. Clarifying your aim/purpose of the study and developing a clear research question will guide your search. Some reasons might include:

- I am a curious person who likes to know why and how things happen.
- I am working in a hospital or other profession, and part of my position includes doing research on hot topics and presenting my findings to the staff.
- I am expected to conduct research as an undergraduate or graduate student assignment.
- This is an integral part of my master's or doctoral program.
- I am.… What is your reason?

The reason why you are embarking on a research project matters because it can help determine the parameters of your research, the time frame you have to conduct the research and report your findings, and the expectations that may exist for publication (yours and others).

Formal research projects need to follow the format established by the institution requiring the research. The process of finding the evidence is similar, but the depth of the inquiry and the format for reporting what you find may vary. This chapter provides a general introduction to the literature review. For those of you involved in formal institutional research, you *must* follow the guidelines of your institution.

If you are working on a thesis, DNP project, or dissertation, the review of the literature will most likely be the second chapter of your report. It will provide support for the argument established in the first chapter (background) and serve as the foundation to launch your own research proposal. The review of the literature establishes the published history of the problem as well as the generally accepted importance of the topic. It is also during the literature review that your topic will be refocused and refined and rewritten, based upon what you find.

Some Mousetraps to Avoid

Overexcitation and Expansion of the Original Idea

Warning! Some new ideas might pop into your head (some of them great ideas, in fact) for changing your research topic during the literature search. This can be overwhelming, and it is best to accept that you will remain focused on the AIM of your project and the research question you have developed. If other ideas do intrude, put them on a different piece of paper for consideration at a later time. More often than not, going off on tangents early in your process might make you feel that you are totally lost. Take heart, you are not lost; you are just off the highway that takes you to your project's end. Get back to your map and you will arrive at your destination.

The old adage "Keep it simple, stupid (KISS)" may have been created to guide new researchers away from frustrations. The more variables you have in your study, the more difficult it will be to determine which, if any, variables are related to each other. If your study includes an experiment in which one variable affects another, too many variables will muddy your results. Think of it like a soup. If we say that adding a pinch of salt to chicken broth improves the flavor, and at the same time we add celery, carrots, and parsley, it is hard to say what, if any, impact the addition of salt has on taste.

Researching Commonly Investigated Topics

When you dive into the existing literature, you might find that your exact topic has already been researched a lot, with the same or different populations. This means that you have chosen a topic that has been of interest to many people. This could be a good thing or not, depending on why you are doing the research. If you are a person doing this research because of your own interest in the topic, your search might be done. You can look over this research and perhaps find the answer to your questions. The same applies to the person who has identified a discrepancy in the workplace. If you find the answer in your literature search, a short report reflective of the existing literature can be used in your committee, or even published. This is different, however, if you've been tasked to conduct, report, and publish original research.

Tips to Help You Refocus After Landing in a Mousetrap

In all cases, however, your first task is to read what you can find about your topic. If during your initial search, you discover that your exact topic has been researched already, you have a choice: either you change the population (or some other variable of the research) to see if the outcome is the same with your population, or you can choose a different topic. If the other research was done a few years ago (like 5+ years), you could still do the research and compare your results to those found in the past.

LITERATURE REVIEW BENEFITS

Getting Value From the Literature Review Experience

Finding Similar Research During Your Literature Review: Modeling

It might happen that the topic you want to research is slightly different from the topics you have found in the review. Or it might turn out that the research reported in one article is close enough to yours that it helps you identify a method that might work for your research. You can use the existing article as a model, demonstrating a way to simplify your question, identifying and explaining how to use an existing public measurement tool, clarifying how to run the experiment, spotlighting how to analyze the data, and maybe even providing you with a method or guide on how to report your findings.

Finding Other References Used by One of the Authors of Research Like Your Own

At the end of each article are references that demonstrate where the researcher got information for the study. These references can be a gold mine for the novice researcher, providing articles, key search words, and new ideas.

As you can see, the benefits of a good review of the literature are multifold. Not only does it identify what has been done, it can also help to clarify possible methods to utilize in future research projects, exposes gaps in current knowledge, and provide models for refining current topics being considered.

WHERE TO START

After the Aim and Research Questions Come Variable Identification, Keywords, and Databases

There are many different ways to start a review of the current litera-ture. This book will identify one way, but it is not the only way; in fact, it is one of many. The review of the literature will be a reflection on the BIG PROBLEM and what has been published before on that topic. It will introduce the current problem as well and be guided by the *aim* and *research question*. Getting into a literature search is somewhat like going on a vacation. When you take a trip, you should know where you want to go, how you want to get there, and how much you have to spend. If you have not considered these things, you might get on the wrong transportation, headed in the wrong direction, costing more than you have, and wondering how it all happened. So, some basic things to consider before starting on your literature search are:

- How far back will you want to go? If this is an historical approach to a problem, your search will be including many more years than if this is one that looks at the trends of the past decade.
- How broad do you want it to be? If your study is about women's health in Florida, the breadth of the search might be much narrower than if you were comparing health initiatives for women in Florida and Canada.

So let us set up, using the formula you have learned in the first three chapters, a research study:

Consider the following news report (Ratterman, 2018) as the current problem that has been identified for your study. The **discrep-ancy** you identify is this: Students in college should be in a safe learn-ing environment, but alcohol-related experiences for students coming back to school have made it unsafe. Current problem: Freshmen drinking alcohol are getting hurt. BIG PROBLEM: Freshmen drink-ing kills some students and can impact the lives of many others.

The AIM of this project is to identify patterns of freshmen drinking
on college campuses, so to start this literature search, the broadest
topic will be *identifying alcohol-drinking patterns of college freshmen*.
Our RESEARCH QUESTION will be "What impacts drinking patterns of college freshmen?"

What Has Been Written on This Topic?

Now comes the task of finding what, if anything, has been written
on the alcohol-drinking patterns of college freshmen students. It is
important that we start to narrow our search already.

Questions to Ask to Narrow Our Search

- What is the BIG PROBLEM, and why are we interested in it?
- How am I defining the elements and variables?
    - What is meant by *patterns*?
    - What is meant by *alcohol*? Is any alcohol considered, or are we
      interested in specific alcohol (beer, wine, spirits)?
    - What is meant by *freshmen*? Is it the typical age group of
      freshmen students, after high school (17–19 years of age) or all
      freshmen?

Good news, once this first set of questions are answered, you have
already narrowed the search a bit! But just like deciding you want to
go on vacation (very broad) to narrowing it down to going on vacation in Florida (less broad) to visiting Orlando (fairly specific), there

is still more to do in order to actually get going on the vacation. It is the same with the literature search. Going slowly, using a process, can help you avoid feeling overwhelmed and can support your identification of what is really important to your study. The first few searches might yield too many articles to consider, but do not lose sight of why you are doing this. You are setting up the argument of the importance of this topic. Refresh your thoughts about why this study is important.

What other items do you think might be helpful in narrowing the focus on this literature review on the patterns of freshmen alcohol drinking? Refine your variables even further! For the trip to Orlando, you might specify where you want to stay, what sights you want to see, and how you want to get there. For the study on patterns of freshmen drinking, you might want to drill down by specifying if you are interested in:

- Students at 4-year or 2-year colleges
- Specific genders
- Specific geographical areas in America
- National or international students

If the topic still seems too broad to you, you can engage in identifying other descriptive traits like:

- Specific students, that is, nursing students, liberal arts students
- Students with English as a second language
- Students who work while going to school

As you can see, the topic of alcohol patterns in college students can become very broad. So unless it is focused in a little, you might get lost in the literature and never make it to Chapter 3, "From Hypothesis to Aim/Purpose," of your report! In order to focus, start with identification of variables (factors) that will be important to your study. Table 4.1 shows two topics broken into variables and categories of interest. *Example in action:* Can you add two more?

Now that you have narrowed the topic, the demographics, and the variables of interest, it is time to refine even further.

REFINE: Starting With the Time Frame

First identify your time frame for the literature search. As you are just embarking on this investigation, you might want to limit the first line of your search to the current year. This will automatically reduce the number of "hits" you will get. As you clarify your variables (like age, type of college, geographical area, gender) and identify other studies that have used similar variables, you can refine your question and expand the years of inquiry included in the search.

Table 4.1

Topics and Variable Identification				
Topic	**Demographic Variable**	**Category**	**Specific Variable of Interest**	**Category**
Student alcohol use	Age	18–21	Type of college	2-year vs. 4-year college
Student study habits	Gender	Female	NCLEX® scores	Passing scores

Table 4.2

Refining a Search by Narrowing Time Frame				
Keywords	**Time Frame**	**Google**	**Google Scholar**	**PubMed**
College drinking	None	474 million	2,879,000	16,025
College drinking	Since 2010	110 million	486,000	10,340
College drinking	2018	103 million	29,000	1,643

Usually you will want to look at articles from the past decade, but more recent articles are better, as a rule of thumb. However, if the research is comparing different periods of time and the healthcare policy of those eras, articles reflective of the information you need would be more beneficial.

Limiting the time frame for published articles can be one method to narrow your search to the most current knowledge on that topic.

Example in action: Refining by narrowing time frame for search (see Table 4.2).

REFINE! Narrowing the Keywords

Now it is time to begin refining your keywords, including only the variables of interest to your study.

Example in action: Refining by narrowing variables of interest and topic-specific search engines (see Table 4.3).

As you can see, the more specified the search engine, the more specific the identification of published articles. For nursing-specific journals, the EBSCO Nursing resource of Cumulative Index to Nursing and Allied Health Literature (CINAHL) is a great place to start. A chart at the end of this chapter lists the specific search engines and their websites, but if you have access to an academic library, see your librarian for those engines you will have access to.

Table 4.3

Refining a Search by Narrowing the Keywords With Variables of Interest: Example in Action				
Keywords	Time Frame	Google	Google Scholar	PubMed
Freshmen college drinking	2018	23.4 million	3,740	7
Female freshmen college drinking	2018	17.5 million	3,200	2
Female freshmen college drinking in Arkansas	2018	1.9 million	1,180	0

REFINE! Using Exact Language

Using language as a tool to refine the search is also possible. You can search most databases for matching exact words simply by adding single quotation marks around the phrase (e.g., 'Freshmen Drinking Behaviors'), which will limit your search to the specific words in the exact order of your specific phrase.

REVIEWING THE ABSTRACT

Each article will have an abstract (a short summary of about 200–250 words). By reviewing the abstract, you will be able to have a good idea what the article is about and if it is relevant to your study.

USING LITERATURE TO FIND MORE LITERATURE

- When you find an article that is very helpful to you in describing the problem, or providing a model that you can follow for your own research, looking at the references used by that author can direct you to other articles that are related to your topic.
- Refer to a citation index: A citation index is a way to find out who has cited the author/article you are interested in. Your school library can assist you to do an electronic search of those authors who are also researching your topic. Remember that not all the articles that you find will be in agreement with the original author's theory or hypothesis. Sometimes an author is referenced in an article because the more recent studies have disputed the original idea.

(continued)

USING LITERATURE TO FIND MORE LITERATURE (*continued*)

■ When there are statistics involved, you might not get the most up-to-date statistics on your topic from an article that is 5 or 6 years old. Looking at where the author found the cited statistics and then going to that database and searching the database for current statistics is a good way to make sure you have the most up-to-date information. Citing older statistics does not strengthen your argument if they lack current validity.

Keeping It Organized

A good way to start your review is to identify a way to keep all the literature organized. You can use existing organization tools (see the end of the chapter for links) or devise your own.

You might find several articles that are of interest to you, and sometimes the more articles you find, the more confused you might get about your "Big Problem" as well as your own research topic. Organizing the articles, and keeping your focus on what your aim and your research question are, can help you focus in on YOUR study.

When you make a table, it is easier to identify which articles are similar to your topic and which ones go in a different direction. You will be able to compare the samples as well as the outcomes. A quick glance at your table will also help distinguish between methods. After you have the articles in your table, you can begin to write up the literature review that compares and contrasts the various articles of interest, giving a synopsis of the articles and identifying if there is a gap that is filled by your study.

Here are some suggestions of different ways to categorize your literature. Some institutions have already decided to work with a specific method for arranging the literature in a review, so check with your institution to determine if a method has already been adopted for use.

The decision of how to store your literature review organizers is up to you. It can be done electronically, using an existing reference app like RefWorks, or the old-fashioned way by printing out the articles and putting them together with the reviews in binders. The important thing is that you know your organization tool and you keep it updated.

Long Reviews

Divide your articles into four categories: literature reviews, qualitative, quantitative, and mixed methods. Write up a small synopsis of your thoughts on the article, include the abstract, and write how this article adds to your background or discussion. If you have cited any sentences, you can either put them in your synopsis with the page number or color-code them with a highlighter, numbering the colors in the long review.

THE LONG REVIEW

Design: Nonexperimental, cross-sectional, survey

Setting: Northeastern public university

Sample: 422 undergraduate freshmen college students

Topic: What, if any, influence does knowledge and attitude toward university policy toward alcohol use have on freshmen students' patterns of drinking?

Findings: Most students had knowledge of policies and consequences of nonadherence to school policies. The knowledge did not impact the behaviors of students participating in the study. As is stated in the theory of planned behavior, the students' attitude toward alcohol use had a greater predictive value than knowledge of school policy.

Quotation: "Strategies include acknowledging and supporting the non-drinking student (i.e., providing alternative drinking activities) and providing accurate information related to the alcohol use social norm. Reducing alcohol use makes the learning environment on a campus safer for all. Methods to reduce alcohol use by students include consistent enforcement of alcohol related policies on campus, provision of non-alcohol events, and comprehensive social norming initiatives" (Marshall, Roberts, Donnelly, & Rutledge, 2011, p. 355).

Source: Marshall, B., Roberts, K., Donnelly, J., & Rutledge, I. (2011). College students perceptions on campus alcohol policies and consumption patterns. *Journal of Drug Education, 41*(4), 345–358. doi:10.2190/DE.41.4.a

Short Reviews

This is explained using a table for research articles (Exhibit 4.1; see link for full article)

Exhibit 4.1

Table Organizing Short Reviews of Research Articles

Author(s) Date Link	Research Question	Sample and Size	Type of Research: Data Collection Method	Data Analysis	Results	Comments
1) Marshall, B., Roberts, K., Donnelly, J., & Rutledge, I. (2011). College students perceptions on campus alcohol policies and consumption patterns. *Journal of Drug Education, 41*(4), 345–358.	What is the role of knowledge and attitude toward alcohol policies on student drinking behavior?	422 college students	Nonexperimental, descriptive, cross-sectional, survey	Univariate analysis and Tukey's honestly significant difference (HSD) post hoc comparisons T-tests	Knowledge of policy did not translate into drinking abstinence.	Supports the theory of planned behavior, taking into consideration student attitudes and intentions as being more indicative of student drinking behaviors.

(continued)

Exhibit 4.1

Table Organizing Short Reviews of Research Articles (*continued*)

Author(s) Date Link	Research Question	Sample and Size	Type of Research: Data Collection Method	Data Analysis	Results	Comments
2) Author ABC. (2019). Title. Journal, volume(issue), pages. (FAKE ARTICLE)	Is alcohol use higher in freshmen or seniors?	20 college students	Qualitative Focus group	Text transcription Theme identification	Seniors reported drinking less than freshmen	The focus group of 10 seniors and 10 freshmen identified some understanding of seniors that those freshmen who drank excessively did not remain in school. Difference in years too great to compare the two articles.

1) **Marshall et al. Abstract:** "Environmental strategies for colleges and universities to reduce alcohol consumption among their students include the development and enforcement of campus alcohol policies. This study examines students' knowledge and attitudes toward campus alcohol policies and how they relate to alcohol consumption and alcohol social norms. A sample of 422 freshman students were surveyed during their first month at a 4-year public college. Findings indicated that the majority of students (89%) were aware of campus policies, yet of those who were aware, less than half (44%) were accepting of these campus rules and regulations. In addition, the majority (79%) of students drank at social events, despite this behavior being in direct violation of campus alcohol policies. However, those who supported campus rules consumed significantly less alcohol at social events than those who opposed or had no opinion of the rules. Also, those who supported the rules perceived that their peers and students in general consumed significantly less alcohol at social events than those who were opposed or had no opinion. This outcome supports the premise established by several theories of behavior change including the theory of planned behavior, which state that behavior is influenced less by knowledge than by attitude and intention."

Link: https://journals.sagepub.com/doi/pdf/10.2190/DE.41.4.a?casa_token=jbzhd-U4HN8AAAAA%3Ayog1st24k-_joROJXHmUyHBoMldrl0t105kOvY6Uwmmokj QAtLhY0-u1bSIAc8lZ6VCmgZadzigA

2) Author ABC (2019) Place the exact abstract here and the link.

GAPS IN THE LITERATURE: FINDING THEM AND REPORTING THEM IN YOUR REVIEW

Your literature review will be highlighting what is found in the current literature about your topic. By organizing your review in such a way that you can see what has been reported, it should also help you to identify what is missing. Finding a gap in the literature allows you to substantiate the merit or importance of your study, which will provide information that might help to fill that gap. For example, using the article cited earlier, the authors explain this in their background: "This study extends the literature by investigating the combination of knowledge about and attitudes toward campus alcohol policies and its relation to alcohol drinking behavior and perceived drinking behaviors of others. The role of the combination of knowledge attitude toward alcohol policies and its relation with drinking behavior and perceived peer and other student drinking norms has not been reported in the literature" (Marshall et al., 2011, p. 349).

Fast Facts

Fake and Unethical Publishers

Yes, fake news has been introduced into scholarly articles. As you dive into the journals, searching for information on your topic, it is important to know that not all the journals are created equally.

A number of articles have clearly identified the problems arising for academics and researchers alike by the proliferation of these predator publications (Beall, 2013; Dadkhah, Maliszewski, & Teixeira da Silva, 2016; Shen & Bjork, 2015; Sorooshian, 2017). This poses multiple dangers for the new researcher.

- Citing information that is incorrect.
- Referencing science that is not based in research or established standards.
- Being wooed by the fake and unethical publishers (FUPs) to pay to publish your work, which will be costly and not yield the respect due a well-crafted study.

Not all open access publishers are predatory, and it is not always evident which publishers are reliable. For the novice researcher, finding articles that are published in respected, known publications in a field is a good place to start. These publications require

(continued)

(continued)

that the authors go through a rigorous blind review (three or more reviewers who are experts in the field) prior to getting their work published.

Pay-to-publish and open access publications have increased the number of journals accepting authors. Unfortunately, publishers that are predatory (FUPS [flawed, uncertain, proximate, sparse]) often engage in fake peer reviews and other deceitful activities, which are dishonest or nonacademic and which make determining what to cite a more difficult endeavor.

When reviewing an article/abstract, check to see:

- Author credentials
- Use of cited primary resources
- Credibility of publication/publisher
- Lack of grammatical and spelling errors in the article

MORE MOUSETRAPS!

Avoiding Another Mousetrap: Never, Always, Truth, Prove, and Facts...

Many new researchers are very passionate about their topics and may slide, inadvertently, into the trap of trying to "prove" their point. Research does not set out to prove; its purpose is to investigate. The world is not a perfect place, and many times there are errors in reporting or limitations in other aspects of research design. When writing up the review of the article, be certain to stay true to the words of the researchers, and avoid the tendency to state a result as a truth or a proven fact.

Fast Facts

Self-Evaluation: Three Topics and Literature Reviews

ABC hospital is applying for Magnet° status, identifying their nursing staff as meeting established standards of excellence. The director of nursing has tasked the units to engage in varying levels of research. One group will look on their units to identify some topic

(continued)

(continued)

that could stand improvement, reflective of delivering transforming care at the bedside (TCAB). The group identified the topic of patient satisfaction related to placing a board in each room with the date and name of the care team.

The second group has been asked to identify aspects of care that are present in the hospital that are believed to be unique to the hospital. This group identified the posthospitalized personalized phone calls from the unit team to the patient within 7 days of discharge.

The third group has identified finding existing research being conducted in the hospital. Their topic is related to newborn weights in the neonatal intensive care unit (NICU). They will be looking at nurses' response to increased parental responsibility for tube feeding.

Group 1: TCAB: chalkboards in patients' rooms
Group 2: Discharge follow-up calls from primary nurses
Group 3: NICU birth weights: nurses' response to more parental responsibility for tube feeding

Choose one of these topics and go through the process of mapping out a review of the literature:

1. State the big problem
2. Identify the current specific topic
3. State the purpose and research question
4. Refine by looking at specific variables and time frames
5. Find five articles and place them in a chart with accompanying short reviews

ROUNDUP

This chapter introduced the review of the literature as an exploration into what is already known about your topic. It guided you to clarification of the problem at hand, the variables of interest, and the specific topic related to your research question. The report you craft from the review of the relevant literature should help the reader logically make the trip from the problem and the aim of your study to the fact that the literature supports the importance of this topic and needs YOUR STUDY to shine the light on some critical missing aspect.

SOME ELECTRONIC DATABASES FOR NURSING, MEDICINE, PUBLIC HEALTH, AND PSYCHOLOGY (WITH LINKS TO INSTRUCTIVE VIDEOS)

How to do a literature review using Google Scholar: https://www.youtube.com/watch?v=8ydzerd9FT0

How to use Google Scholar to find journal articles | Essay tips: https://www.youtube.com/watch?v=dc-vKk205c8

How to use ProQuest: https://www.youtube.com/watch?v=d2KLaQulgFA

Literature searching using the PICO method: https://www.youtube.com/watch?v=WPCYqb2pkU0

PICO searches in CINAHL (Cumulative Index to Nursing and Allied Health Literature): https://www.youtube.com/watch?v=-KPyuenYdlg

PsycARTICLES tutorial: https://www.youtube.com/watch?v=I_Y7HVdH1TQ

Searching PsycINFO (on the Ovid Platform): https://www.youtube.com/watch?v=5o3kB0X8K7g

Quick tips & shortcuts for database searching: https://www.youtube.com/watch?v=aWqdF9L4D24

If you are part of an academic environment, visit your school library online and click on databases, reference library, or help desk to determine which online databases you have access to.

LINKS TO LEARN MORE

Fake vs. real: Identifying & evaluating information sources: Fake scholarly articles: http://researchguides.smu.edu.sg/c.php?g=732802&p=5240669

How to write a literature review: https://www.youtube.com/watch?v=rnHvO5aRXq0

Literature review chart: https://visualization.sites.clemson.edu/reu/ResearchMethods/LiteratureReviewTemplate_Part1.pdf

References

Beall, J. (2013). Medical publishing triage-chronicling predatory open access publishers. *Annals of Medicine and Surgery, 2*(2), 47–49. doi:10.1016/S2049-0801(13)70035-9

Dadkhah, M., Maliszewski, T., & Teixeira da Silva, J. (2016). Hijacked journals, hijacked web-sites, journal phishing, misleading metrics, and predatory publishing: Actual and potential threats to academic integrity and publishing ethics. *Forensic Science, Medicine and Pathology, 12*, 353–362. doi:10.1007/s12024-016-9785-x

Marshall, B., Roberts, K., Donnelly, J., & Rutledge, I. (2011). College student perceptions on campus alcohol policies and consumption patterns. *Journal of Drug Education, 41*(4), 345–358. doi:10.2190/DE.41.4.a

Ratterman, R. (2018). Miami students' first weekend back on campus brings spike in alcohol-related emergency calls. *Journal-News.* Retrieved from https://www.journal-news.com/news/crime--law/miami-students-first-weekend-back-campus-brings-spike-alcohol-related-emergency-calls/OGNGrGUbJS8Qts8FbuvZXJ

Shen, C., & Bjork, B. C. (2015). 'Predatory' open access: A longitudinal study of article volumes and market characteristics. *BMC Medicine, 13,* 230. doi:10.1186/s12916-015-0469-2

Sorooshian, S. (2017). Scholarly black market. *Science and Engineering Ethics, 23,* 623–624. doi:10.1007/s11948-016-9765-2

5

The Theoretical Framework

INTRODUCTION, or *Finding the scaffolding: The theoretical framework*

This chapter is devoted to examining the theoretical framework. The theoretical framework can provide structure to the research project, like using a blueprint from another home that closely resembles the one you would like to construct and also identifies the important elements of the place you want to live in. It can provide a philosophical as well as a methodological model to follow while considering what kind of study you will conduct, what design fits your study, and ultimately what kinds of data you will want to collect.

OBJECTIVES

In this chapter you will learn:

- The usefulness of theories
- To identify concepts and constructs in a theory
- The purpose of a theoretical framework
- How to identify a theoretical framework that can be a good fit for your study

IMPORTANT DEFINITIONS

Some of the important vocabulary for this chapter includes the following:

Theory: Put most simply, a theory is an explanation that describes some phenomenon. Theories are developed by observing the phenomenon, collecting data on it, analyzing the data, and then retesting it (experimentation) to see if the outcome is the same. In this way the explanation or theory that evolves is based in scientific process.

Hypothesis: A hypothesis is an explanation or prediction of a phenomenon but is not based upon data. It provides the jumping off point for further investigation of the phenomenon.

Concept: A concept is an abstract idea of something that can be described in a way that makes it identifiable as a separate entity with its own meaning when it stands alone (Shaffer, Sandau, & Missal, 2017). It makes up the most basic component in a theory.

Construct: The term *construct* in research indicates a broader aspect of the theory, one that can combine multiple concepts in it. The construct reflects characteristics; it has a clear definition with a capacity to measure the elements that define it.

Theoretical Framework: This framework will identify the concepts and constructs being studied according to the model or theory it is based in. If the project is not being conducted around an existing theory or model, the framework is referred to as a conceptual, rather than theoretical, framework.

Model: Research models usually demonstrate the relationship that exists between concepts and constructs. Unlike the theories, models are not considered to be as rigorously tested as theories.

Nursing Theories: Nursing theory has been defined as a method to combine and test concepts providing a systematic and purposeful way of viewing nursing phenomena (Chinn & Kramer, 2011). These theories specifically focus on events intrinsic and important to the profession of nursing. Some nursing theories are the need theory (Henderson), the unitary human beings theory (Rogers), the self-care theory (Orem), and the interpersonal theory (Peplau).

Theories on Behavior and Social Norms: Social and behavioral theories, not unlike nursing theories, evolve from the examination and testing of concepts and constructs related to behavior change and are often used in public health projects. These theories seek to predict and/or explain human behaviors under certain circumstances. Some behavioral theories are the Health Belief Model (Hochbaum, Rosenstock, and Kegels), the Transtheoretical Model and Stages of Change (Prochaska and DiClemente), the Theory of Planned Behavior (TPB; Ajzen and Fishbein), and the Social Cognitive Theory (Bandura).

THEORETICAL FRAMEWORK BASICS

If you are considering building a home, you might be looking at other homes that are close representations of your dream home. In addition to the actual house you are building, there are other considerations that would identify a dream home. The guideline or map you might follow to find the elements of the dream home would include some ideas of where you want to live and some clear, measurable indicators of community well-being. For example, you might consider the neighborhoods, the schools, the taxes, and the building costs of similar houses, important elements of the place you want to build a home. This mapping can help guide you toward clarifying and measuring those factors considered relevant to building your home in a good, welcoming, and affordable neighborhood. Without taking these things into consideration, even though you build the best home you can, if you have not understood those important variables, your home might become a nightmare, not the dream home you had anticipated.

Theoretical frameworks are like the guidelines in the preceding example. They establish the important variables that should be measured and, in some cases, even describe how to measure them. The framework is the scaffolding that helps the researcher put together a research design (see Chapter 6, "Research Design") that will provide answers to the question at hand, but it also helps relate to the broader problem under scrutiny (the BIG PROBLEM).

Like building the house, you might have the best architect and plans (research design), but if you have not looked at the specific phenomenon that you consider to be a livable neighborhood (a measurable construct) and assessed the variables that make up that construct as defined and proved by others before you (a theoretical framework), attaining your goal could be undermined by unexpected challenges.

It pays to stand on the shoulders of the giants that have come before us! The theoretical framework is our research map—a map drawn by brilliant cartographers, identifying relationships between variables and outcomes when set in specific circumstances. Just like the novice traveler, without using a map, it is easy to get lost. If we do not know where we are going, it is impossible to even identify the map we will need. So, we start with the BIG PROBLEM, the discrepancy, the specific problem, and the question that we want to research. From there we go to the literature, to see what is already known about our topic. In that search of the literature, we will find a number of maps that can guide us toward creating a study that will help us find some answers to our question. It is as easy as that. Too often, in studying research methods, the vocabulary of research can become confusing and interfere with the understanding that this process, like building a house or going on a trip, needs to be done with thoughtfulness, clarity of purpose, and good decision-making.

THEORIES

In Chapter 1, "Introduction to Research," we discussed the scientific process. It is through the scientific process that theories are established. Theorists, those who develop the theories, are masters of collecting ideas, analyzing content, and clarifying conclusions, and they do so using a method of cogent reasoning (Mithaug, 2000). The resulting theories provide explanations about our world. These theories have undergone testing and retesting and have been demonstrated to be credible (believable) and valuable through establishing coherence, which is backed by logic, validity, and verifiability. So why does this tend to get so confusing? Let's break it down and make it specific.

USING THE BUTTON TO CHANGE THE CROSSING LIGHT

Recently there have been a large number of fatal accidents on Main and Sprain Streets during rush hour, related to the nonuse of a crosswalk change button. If pedestrians push the button, the traffic will stop and allow them to cross the street. The software shows that the button is rarely being pushed in the mornings between 7 and 9 a.m. and the evenings between 4 and 6 p.m. Over the past 2 months, because pedestrians are not using the button, the number of people getting killed at this intersection has greatly risen.

BIG PROBLEM: Death while crossing a busy street.

Discrepancy: There is a crosswalk button that can change the light and let the pedestrian cross safely, but people are not using the button and are getting killed.

(continued)

USING THE BUTTON TO CHANGE THE CROSSING LIGHT (*continued*)

Current Problem: Increased fatalities on the corner of Main and Sprain Streets.

Aim/Purpose: To identify why people are not using the crosswalk button. (Remember, there can be multiple aims or purposes for this kind of study, but for now it will be this one.)

Research Question: Why are pedestrians at Main and Sprain not using the crosswalk button during rush hour?

The hypothesis in the preceding case is this: *If pedestrians used the crosswalk button, then there would be fewer fatalities at Main Street and Sprain Street.*

Now the researchers need to conduct their literature review. In doing so they come up with a number of studies related to safe behavior and road crossings. Three of these studies will be presented here. The first article they find that is of particular interest to them is a study by Hemmati and Gharlipour (2017). It focuses on middle school children and injury due to motor vehicle accidents when crossing the street. This article provides the researchers with a number of similar circumstances and introduces possible important factors, including a possible *theoretical framework*:

1. It provides a background literature review, identifying 14 other articles that deal with the same subject.
2. It identifies a method for data collection.
3. It identifies a theory (TPB) to explain the phenomenon of unsafe crossings.

There are a number of things, however, this article *does not* do. For example, it uses a different subject group (middle schoolers), and it does not identify the use of buttons for changing the crossing light and improving safety.

The second investigation, "Overview of Pedestrian Crash Countermeasures and Safety Programs" in a government study entitled *A Review of Pedestrian Safety Research in the United States and Abroad* (Campbell, Zegeer, Huang, & Cynecki, 2004), provides some clarity on pedestrian behavior and use of crosswalk buttons, as well as alternatives to improve pedestrian safety. It provides the researchers with multiple theories on pedestrian accidents related to human behavior.

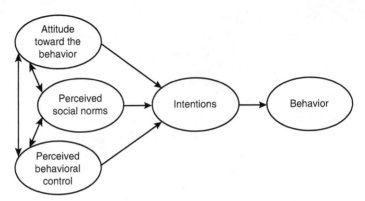

Figure 5.1 Theory of planned behavior: Ajzen's model of planned behavior.
Source: Ajzen, I. (1991). The theory of planned behavior. *Organizational Behavior and Human Decision Processes, 50*, 179–211. doi:10.1016/0749-5978(91)90020-T

The third article discusses the illusion of control (Gino, Sharek, & Moore, 2011) and a person's behavioral intention based upon the psychology of personal control. This article demonstrates how a person's perception of success at doing something impacted his or her actual behavior of engagement. It reinforces TPB as a method for explaining why people engage in specific behaviors. After the review of the literature, it is time for the researchers to make a decision on a framework and a choice on how to go forward with their study.

The researchers decide that they want to use TPB as their framework (Ajzen, 1991; see Figure 5.1). Their review of the literature shifts to focus specifically on the chosen theoretical framework and helps them toward clarification of elements of their study as they might fit into the constructs of TPB. This review helps them to determine that this is the right framework for them, as it has been demonstrated to be predictive in multiple settings related to human behavior and intentions.

CONCEPTS AND CONSTRUCTS

Identifying Concepts and Constructs in a Theory

TPB includes the concept of self-efficacy, or a person's belief in an ability to be successful at a behavior or experience, as presented by Bandura (1982). Theories, like research studies, use the work of those before them to help clarify and test hypotheses so that a cogent, valid, valuable theory can be developed.

The constructs identified in TPB include behavioral intention, attitude toward the behavior, the subjective norm, and perceived behavioral control. Behavioral intention refers to a person's motivation to do something. The more motivated a person is, the more likely the person will intend on completing the behavior. The second, attitude about the behavior, tests how the person feels about the specific behavior. If there is a negative feeling toward that behavior, the person is less likely to want to engage in it. The third one, or subjective norm, refers to the pressure of others to engage. If it is what everyone is doing (their social norm), then there might be pressure for the person to adopt the behavior as a personal (subjective) norm. The final construct of perceived control examines how difficult the person considers the behavior to be. The higher the difficulty, the lower the likelihood of wanting to attempt the behavior.

Now that the theoretical framework has been chosen, it is important for the researchers to consider how they will quantify or measure the constructs that will predict the targeted behavior. Fishbein and Ajzen (2010) identify a method called TACT (target, action, context, and time).

Fast Facts

Spotlight on Theory of Planned Behavior and
Target, Action, Context, and Time

Who is the target in the study? People who use the crosswalk.
What is the action of interest? Pushing the button.
What is the context? When crossing Main and Strain Streets.
What is the time? Rush hour.

Source: Fishbein, M., & Ajzen, I. (2010). *Predicting and changing behavior: The reasoned action approach*. New York, NY: Psychology Press.

The identification of the theoretical framework, as a result of a well-crafted research problem and subsequent literature search, has helped the researchers clarify what they need to look for, what they want to evaluate, and the constructs of interest that could help answer their research question of "Why are pedestrians at Main and Sprain not using the crosswalk button during rush hour?" The researchers still have a way to go before they can start their project, but now they have identified the important factors that might shed light on the problem.

Identifying a Theoretical Framework That Can Be a Good Fit for Your Study

As was demonstrated in the preceding example with the crosswalk buttons, the first step to getting started on your study will be to identify the problem, the big problem, and the discrepancy. Following the process for successful research projects helps the researcher avoid some of the common problems and pitfalls. The clearer the problem, aim, and research question, the more focused the search in the literature will be. Keeping the attention of the search on similar past research can help to define what the specific problem needing an answer is. That literature search will present the researcher with multiple theoretical frameworks to choose from; it is the role of the researcher to be clear on which one will shed the most light on the problem at hand.

Now it is your turn. Before considering how to go about collecting your data, or even what data you need to collect, take some time to think about the problem, the aim, and the research question. See if you are able to fill in the information in the Fast Facts about clarifying problem, aim, and research question.

NURSING THEORIES AND MODELS

The profession of nursing has many theorists whose theories have guided nursing education and practice derived from the science of nursing. "Nursing Science, a basic science, is the substantive discipline specific knowledge that focuses on the human-universe-health process articulated in the nursing frameworks and theories. The discipline-specific knowledge resides within schools of thought that reflect differing philosophical perspectives that give rise to ontological, epistemological, and methodological processes for the development and use of knowledge concerning nursing's unique phenomenon of concern" (Parse et al., 2000, p. 177). Nursing theory reflects the body of work that nursing scholars have developed that is specific to the implementation of the nursing process to embrace nursing philosophies and reflect the focus nursing places on the whole person.

Fast Facts

Clarifying Problem, Aim, and Research Question; Constructing the Literature Search; Identifying a Theoretical Framework

CURRENT PROBLEM:_____
DISCREPANCY:_____
BIG PROBLEM: _____
AIM/PURPOSE:_____
QUESTION:_____

(continued)

(continued)

Literature Review:
Identify topics related to the big problem: keywords?
Identify topics related to the current problem: keywords?
Establish the time frame for review (historical or current—past 10 years).
Identification of possible theoretical frameworks:
1)
2)
3+?
Choose from frameworks one that best aligns itself with your current problem and provides a possible map toward identifying explanations.

Identify constructs and variables as indicated by the framework that need to be clarified and measured.

ROUNDUP

Identifying the theoretical framework for a study should be a result of carefully following the problem at hand through to the development of a clear research question that can be investigated in the literature. The framework will provide the road map for developing a design (see Chapter 6, "Research Design") that will be appropriate for the study, and which will provide some explanations for the existing discrepancy. In each step of this process, it is important to focus on *that* step with clarity and attention. Once you have been able to identify the framework, you will be able to begin the work of singling out the design and the variables and construct your plan of research specific to your problem under scrutiny.

LINKS TO LEARN MORE

How to support research with theoretical and conceptual frameworks: https://www.youtube.com/watch?v=j2c8G0bBfHk
What is a concept? What is a construct? https://www.youtube.com/watch?v=Hdk-8BC86A8

References

Ajzen, I. (1991). The theory of planned behavior. *Organizational Behavior and Human Decision Processes, 50,* 179–211. doi:10.1016/0749-5978(91)90020-T

Bandura, A. (1982). Self-efficacy mechanism in human agency. *American Psychologist, 37*(2), 122–147. doi:10.1037/0003-066X.37.2.122

Campbell, B. J., Zegeer, C. V., Huang, H. H., & Cynecki, M. J. (2004). *A Review of Pedestrian Safety Research in the United States and Abroad* (pp. 57–120). McLean VA: Office of Safety Research and Development, Federal Highway Administration.

Chinn, P., & Kramer, M. (2011). *Integrated theory & knowledge development in nursing* (8th ed.). St. Louis, MO: Mosby.

Fishbein, M., & Ajzen, I. (2010). *Predicting and changing behavior: The reasoned action approach.* New York, NY: Psychology Press.

Gino, F., Sharek, Z., & Moore, D. A. (2011). Keeping the illusion of control under control: Ceilings, floors, and imperfect calibration. *Organizational Behavior and Human Decision Processes, 114*(2), 104–114. doi:10.1016/j.obhdp.2010.10.002

Hemmati, R., & Gharlipour, Z. (2017). Study of the safe behavior in road crossing using the theory of planned behavior among middle school students. *International Journal of Pediatrics, 5*(5), 5003–5012. Retrieved from http://jip.mums.ac.ir

Moithaug, D. E. (2000). *Learning to theorize: A four step strategy.* Thousand Oaks: SAGE.

Parse, R. R., Barrett, E. A. M., Bourgeois, M., Dee, V., Egan, E., Germain, C., … Wolf, G. (2000). Nursing theory-guided practice: A definition. *Nursing Science Quarterly, 13*, 177. doi:10.1177/08943180022107474

Schaffer, M., Sandau, K., & Missal, B. (2017). Demystifying nursing theory: A Christian nursing perspective. *Journal of Christian Nursing, 34*(2), 102–107. doi:10.1097/CNJ.0000000000000375

6

Research Design

Tom Heinzen

INTRODUCTION, or *The mental mechanics of clear thinking*

This chapter examines the importance of the design of your research project. It underscores the concept that the research process is an exercise in clear thinking, which, when done correctly, sheds new light on a problem, question, or theory.

OBJECTIVES

In this chapter you will learn:

- To recognize common threats to good research designs
- The elements of research design
- Strategies of organizing participants in a study
- Common symbols used in a research design
- Different kinds of research designs

IMPORTANT DEFINITIONS

Some of the important vocabulary for this chapter includes the following:

Research Design: The design of your study is like the architect's blueprint. It reflects the clear thinking method to start the construction of an investigation. The design is important to have before the study begins, because you would not want to start building unless you knew that the resulting structure would be solid and safe.

Validity: The validity of a research project reflects not only the fact that the design will measure those factors of importance but also the fact that the method chosen for the study will be appropriate.

Reliability: Another word for *reliability* is *consistency*. Will you get a consistent outcome if you repeat an action over and over? The researcher needs to be able to believe the outcomes are consistent because they are correct measurement, not something arrived at by luck.

Threat: A threat in research design refers to anything that could affect the reliability or validity of the study's outcomes. Different kinds of threats are discussed in this chapter.

Placebo Effects/Expectation Effects: This is the impact that an expectation can have on an experience; although there might be no actual intervention, the person involved experiences a change because there is an expectation of change. Placebo effects are often seen in medication trials, when a patient receiving the placebo, or nonintervention medication, experiences a positive outcome anyway.

Correlation: Correlation in research indicates a relationship between two or more factors. There is sometimes confusion around the notion of correlation, thinking that because two elements are related, there might be a causal relationship. It is important to remember correlation does not imply causation.

Preexperiments: These observations are made without the benefit of scientific controls. They are easily conducted but are not conducted with scientific rigor, and they should not be considered true experiments.

True Experiments: These rigorously designed experiments establish cause and effect through the controlling of variables (intervention and nonintervention groups), manipulating variables, and random assignment of subjects. True experiments are difficult to conduct and are usually done in the lab where the researcher has increased control of the variables and the subjects.

Quasi-Experiment: This design incorporates the use of intervention and nonintervention groups, but as it is conducted in the real world, it usually lacks true random assignment of the subjects.

NAVIGATING PAST THE THREATS TO RESEARCH DESIGN

Applied researchers in the health sciences enjoy privileged opportunities to apply research designs because they work directly with the populations that interest them. However, those opportunities for realism also are laced with threats so subtle and poisonous that they can cause harm rather than healing. We can navigate past these threats only if we are guided by (1) the humility to recognize our own impulses toward confirmation bias and (2) an intimate knowledge of research designs. It's pleasant, of course, to see your name on some publication, to become part of the official community of scientific researchers. But especially with research in the health sciences, we want to be careful. Sometimes the stakes are high.

Fast Facts

Learning About Research Design

The first principle is that you must not fool yourself—and you are the easiest person to fool. So you have to be very careful about that. After you've not fooled yourself, it's easy not to fool other scientists. You just have to be honest in a conventional way after that.

—Physicist Richard Feynman's (1974)
warning to his students

A Case Study of Bad Science by a Good Man

It is easy to admire Dr. Benjamin Rush. He was a signer of the Declaration of Independence and the father of modern psychiatry. In the 1700s, Rush had "served tirelessly as an advocate for many social reforms including temperance, women's rights, and humane treatment of the mentally ill...women's education and the abolition of slavery" (Toledo, 2004, pp. 61–62). Rush was a product of the Enlightenment and, in the United States, decades ahead of his time (see Heinzen & Goodfriend, 2019, p. 4). But even such a fine, well-educated public servant can be victimized by *confirmation bias*, or proving a hypothesis instead of investigating it, as is demonstrated in the following story.

The Story of Dr. Benjamin Rush

Dr. Benjamin Rush believed in heroic medicine—the idea that a desperate illness called for desperate measures. And the desperate measures he advocated during the yellow fever outbreak in Philadelphia in 1793 were bloodletting and purging. Horacio Toledo (2004) tells the story: "Typically, Rush would 'relieve' his patients of eight pints of blood over two or three days" (p. 61). And if that did not work, Rush would administer "another round of bleeding and purging" (p. 61; leeches, cutting, vomiting, and elimination). Get all that bad stuff out of your system! There had been no tests of these well-known methods because their benefits were so obvious and the logic so plain. Rush noticed that many of his extremely ill patients did not die after bloodletting, and that seemed to be all the proof he needed.

Benjamin Rush demonstrated his own personal heroism by bravely applying his theory to the sick people struggling through Philadelphia's contagious yellow fever epidemic. But heroic commitment, sincere belief, and an intuitively appealing theory still did not make his treatment effective. "Without doubt," Toledo concluded, the "brand of heroic medicine initiated and propagated by Rush cost thousands of American lives including his own" (p. 61).

Common Threats to Good Research Designs

The many threats to scientific reasoning include the well-known (but still subtle) *placebo effects* and *expectation effects*. Health science researchers are familiar with these threats; drug companies are required to conduct randomized, double-blind research that controls for placebo effects. These are more than technical requirements because they all are related to the peculiar human frailty that "believing is seeing." Benjamin Rush had also fallen victim to *confirmation bias*, the tendency to pay attention only to evidence that supports what he already believed and to ignore any contradicting evidence.

Less well known is the problem of *regression to the mean* when, for example, what looks like a positive reaction to a treatment is just the normal fluctuation of a disease returning to its healthy baseline. Another naturally occurring threat that can masquerade as an apparent success (and failure) is *maturation*, such as growing older, hungrier, or more fatigued. *Testing effects* (also called *order effects*) are also a threat because taking one test can influence performance when taking the same test for a second time. *Testing/order effects* are harmful when they confound the logic of an experiment, but they are so powerful that they can be turned to positive purposes.

An often-overlooked threat to clear thinking enforced by appropriate research designs is the problem of *response bias*. If you distribute a survey in order to study what motivates physicians, you face a host of threats to clear thinking. The first is probably the problem of *social desirability*, providing slightly dishonest responses in order to protect reputation, provide what they know society wants, or more subtly report what they think the researcher is looking for. Not far behind social desirability is the problem of *self-selection*. Only certain types of physicians will fill out and return the survey. It is difficult to accurately interpret data already biased by who was—and was not— supplying the data.

Fast Facts

What Do You Think?

Mr. Jones is a patient admitted to the unit with an elevated blood pressure (BP). On admission his reading was 180/90. The next morning it was 178/88, at lunch it was 170/90, and that afternoon, after a compassionate nurse spent several minutes listening sympathetically to Mr. Jones, his BP was 140/74.

- Did the nurse's sympathy do the trick?
- Or was BP likely to return to its average on its own (regression to the mean), with or without sympathetic listening?
- Could there be other reasons for the BP to go down?

What do you think?

Lurking beneath these threats to clear thinking is the misperception we can refer to as the *correlation confusion*. As we process our surrounding world, we often assume that two things that co-occur must be causally related. This is a particularly tough weed to remove from our mental garden plots because, although correlation does not imply causation, correlation often really is causation. We flip light switches, press TV remotes, turn car keys, and—voila!—they turn on. Although we repeatedly experience different light switches, televisions, and automobiles, the positive correlations persist. We also constantly assume that correlation implies causation in the health sciences. We administer aspirin, inject a narcotic, or administer exercises for bad knees, and—*voila!*—the patient experiences relief.

Our brains begin analyses with a strong, automatic, and understandable bias to believe that correlation implies causation.

When you combine our fondness for self-serving self-deceptions (see Trivers, 2011) with the correlation confusion, it is easy to understand why Benjamin Rush perceived a positive correlation between bloodletting and recovery from yellow fever. But it was an *illusory correlation*, merely a perceived connection that was deadly to thousands of now long-forgotten lives. The correlation confusion is related logically to the problem of *confounding variables*, co-occurring influences that logically compete with the real cause to explain any apparent correlations.

The nurse might understandably be biased to believe in the effectiveness of his or her own caring compassion. That assumption may be correct, but we will never know—and neither will the nurse—no matter how strongly he or she believes in the power of his or her own compassion. Remember, Benjamin Rush risked his own life because he was so certain about the positive benefits of bloodletting.

Sincerity is an untrustworthy guide to truth.

These are just a few of the many temptations to bias a study in favor of our own hypotheses. They all have useful descriptive names, but the underlying problem is our impulse to believe what is flattering rather than what is real. Fortunately, our knowledge of the weaknesses and strengths of research designs limits our access to the many self-serving, self-deceiving temptations to arrange the evidence to confirm only what we already believe.

THE ELEMENTS OF RESEARCH DESIGNS

The elements of a good research design are the practical guidelines for clear thinking. They are not uniquely scientific because they apply to baking bread, reasoning about human relationships, career decisions, and vaccines. Reliability and validity, for example, are merely practical ways of discovering whether we can trust the recipe for banana bread, the developing romantic relationship, the new boss, or the measles vaccine. The scientific principles that expose bad designs and support good designs are the mental mechanics that describe how humans have learned to think clearly.

Introducing Reliability and Validity

Reliability is a necessary element of clear thinking because it refers to the kind of consistency that is important to a bus schedule or a blood pressure reading. If blood pressure is stable, then a blood pressure reading that varies wildly is a useless measure. Even if the readings are occasionally accurate, the clinician does not know which reading to believe.

There are several subtypes of reliability, or practical ways that we can assess reliability. *Test–retest reliability* is simply repeating a particular blood pressure test to check for consistency. *Inter-rater reliability* compares the judgments between two or more raters assessing blood pressure, to see if they are consistent. *Internal consistency reliability* compares items within an assessment, such as a depression inventory or a concussion symptom checklist, to see if the internal measurements are consistently telling the same story.

Reliability is a necessary but insufficient indicator of how much you can trust your data. But reliability by itself is like rowing a boat with only one side oar. Here's the problem: Your blood pressure readings, like a bus that always leaves 5 minutes early, might be reliable— but reliably wrong!

Validity refers to whether you are measuring what you intended to measure. A reliable presurgery report might indicate that the patient has been properly prepped for surgery. But that will not stop the surgical team from amputating the wrong leg.

There are several subtypes of validity, or practical ways that we can assess validity. *Face validity* asks the obvious question: Does a particular test, on its face, appear to be measuring what it is supposed to measure? A patient expecting a food preference survey (probably) will recognize that a symptom checklist for Alzheimer's disease is invalid. That same scale will also lack *content validity* because the items on the symptom checklist will not be connected to a preference for chocolate or vanilla pudding. *Predictive validity* asks a more demanding question: Are your data predicting what they were supposed to predict? A physical therapist who informs a patient to expect full recovery in 3 to 4 days probably is taking a foolish risk. The prediction will not be valid if the actual recovery is well outside that time window.

Validity depends on reliability. The bus has to be consistent *and* on time. We can only make scientific progress if we can row with two oars: reliability *and* validity. The concepts of reliability and validity as well as their importance in research studies are explored deeply in Chapter 9, "Reliability and Validity."

Strategies for Organizing Participants in a Study

Between-Groups Versus Within-Groups Designs

There are two general strategies for organizing the participants in a study. A *between-groups design* divides study participants into groups, hopefully by using random assignment. Of course, a study comparing males with females cannot use random assignment to sex! However it is achieved, the participants in a between-groups design will belong to an exclusive group. If you are in one group, then you cannot belong to the other group. Imagine that an occupational therapist wants to increase compliance by testing three motivational apps against a control group, with 50 randomly assigned participants in each of the four groups. That study would require 200 total participants.

A *within-groups design* uses the same people for every level of the experiment. That study could succeed with only 50 participants. Participants in the study would report their motivation without any apps and then continue to report their motivation as they experience all three apps. There are distinct advantages and disadvantages to each approach. One obvious advantage of within-groups designs is that they are less expensive if you are paying the participants. A major disadvantage of the within-groups design is testing/order effects, when taking one test influences how well you perform when taking the same test for a second time. Once you have experienced one app, it may well influence your motivational response to the next two apps.

A Note About Symbols

Most of the notations in this chapter will become apparent to you as you examine each type of design. This summary supplies a reference for when you get confused. We cannot improve on the symbolic notation used by Campbell and Stanley (1966), or the descriptions of types of research designs. Our only addition is to identify observations of a stand-alone case study by a solitary symbol: O.

An X represents exposure to some experimental variable or event. O represents some observation. The Xs and Os presented in a row describe specific persons. The left-to-right ordering indicates the passage of time. Xs and Os that are vertically aligned are therefore simultaneous. The letter R indicates random assignment to different treatment groups in order to make all participants equivalent before the experiment begins. When symbols are presented in parallel rows, unseparated by dashes, they represent comparison groups made equal through randomization. Symbols separated by a dashed line represent comparison groups that have not been made equal through random assignment.

TYPES OF RESEARCH DESIGNS

There are three general categories of research designs: preexperiments, true experiments, and quasi-experiments. We provide examples of each category of design.

Preexperiments are easy to conduct and frequently used in applied settings, but they are seldom helpful and occasionally dangerous. True experiments are usually more difficult (and expensive) to conduct in an applied setting, but they are more helpful. Quasi-experiments occupy the middle ground that allows privileged access to special populations by limiting confounds while acknowledging the common threats to good research. If you can find the flaws in each of these research designs, then you will be well on your way to selecting the strongest design that will yield the most reliable answer to your particular research question.

Preexperiments

Preexperiments are observations without the benefit of scientific controls. Four such commonly used but deeply flawed designs are the case study, the one-shot case study, the one-group pretest–posttest design, and the static-group comparison. The most basic preexperiment is the case study, and it is probably the most trustworthy preexperiment but for a strange reason. The case study makes no pretense at being a controlled experiment. You need to be extremely cautious about believing the results of any preexperiment because there is no meaningful comparison group. The absence of a meaningful comparison group invites self-deceptive, self-serving interpretations of data.

Case Studies

A one-time observation may be represented by:

O

A case study is a detailed description of a one-time-only observation, usually of a complex phenomenon. In spite of their lack of scientific controls, case studies have significantly shaped the growth of science (see Rolls, 2015), even when those case studies were the result of accidents. For example, the history of neuroscience owes a debt to the railroad foreman Phineas Gage (see Macmillan, 2002). In 1848, Gage had a 43-inch pointed iron rod explode upward beneath his left cheek, behind his left eye, pierce his skull, and land some 25 feet away covered with his brain matter.

Gage lived, but his once self-controlled personality had changed into an impulsive, often crude individual who, curiously, seemed to have no concept of money. On the other hand, Gage was still able to recognize people, drive a multihorse stage coach, and tell entertaining stories to his nieces and nephews. The fascination with Phineas Gage is twofold: His personality changed, but he remained a capable, functioning individual—with some notable deficits. The problem with such dramatic case studies is that they cannot be easily replicated. Researchers are left to blend his story into emerging scientific knowledge (Dolan, 2007). In terms of design, case studies make great stories, and that makes them even more dangerous. They are so memorable that people attach their own private meanings and accept as scientific fact something that may not be true or is misunderstood.

The One-Shot Case Study Design

The untrustworthy but occasionally unavoidable one-shot case study design can be represented by:

$$X\ O$$

This design moves only a little closer to the ideal true experiment. In this case, something happens before the observation. The seductive but illogical belief is that whatever happened first necessarily caused the observation. For example, I have moved a few times in my career, and the professional sports teams in those cities soon won their championships. Did I cause one team to win the Super Bowl, another to win the World Series, and another to win the Stanley Cup? No. It is more plausible that a key player may have contributed to those successes, but we still cannot experimentally assert that my geographical moves, a particular football quarterback, baseball pitcher, or hockey goalie caused a championship.

For example, imagine that you wanted to test whether hospital patients' satisfaction with meals increased after hiring a new director. A one-shot case study might distribute a survey (sometimes sarcastically called a "smile sheet" by researchers) asking questions loaded with *demand characteristics* that cue participants how the director wants participants to respond. A gross example is, "On a scale of 1 through 5, how happy were you when food was delivered hot and on time?" There might be very different ratings had they asked, "How often was your food delivered hot and on time?"

The One-Group Pretest–Posttest Design

The slightly better but far from perfect one-group pretest–posttest design may be represented by:

$$O_1\ X\ O_2$$

This common preexperimental design, often called a *before–after design*, looks seductively like an experiment. But it is only a little more trustworthy than a one-shot observation. This design is convenient and relatively easy to conduct, and that is a strength that is welcome in the real world of research. However, you must be cautious about believing these results! The silent assumption is that the pretest caused any changes in the posttest. That may or may not be true; we cannot tell.

For example, if hospital management implements a new computer program for progress notes in the ED and then discovers that their billings increase, they will be tempted to credit the new software. However, there are countless potential confounding variables in this design. There may be a new, effective data manager working behind the scenes, the ED may have seasonal fluctuations that are the real cause of any changes in billings, or a nearby ED may have opened or closed. If you do not control for co-occurring events, then you are inviting self-serving misinterpretations that lead you to believe something that is not true.

The Static-Group Comparison

This common, but still uncertain, design would look like this:

$$X \quad O_1$$
$$-------------$$
$$O_2$$

This design is common because it recognizes the need for a meaningful comparison group. However, it does not provide a meaningful comparison group. Imagine, for example, that a health researcher wanted to know whether a 30-minute training workshop influenced scores on an Attitude Toward Patients Scale. So, the researcher compared a hospital that had supplied their nurses with that training (the X) with a hospital without that requirement.

Do you see the problem? The dotted line tells us that the two groups were not created by random assignment. Then how were they created? The answer is usually related to the problem of *self-selection*. Different kinds of nurses will be attracted to hospital 1 and hospital 2. But that's only one of many confounds that may be upsetting the logic of this study. One hospital may be in a rural area and the other in a city. The two hospitals may differ in size, the maturity of their administrators, demographics of the patient population, and the quality of their physical plant. The researcher cannot infer that the cause of any differences in attitudes toward patients was related to the workshop. Our human inclination for self-serving self-deceptions probably will not stop many poorly trained administrators from claiming credit for data that support their hypothesis and finding procedural problems when data do not support that hypothesis. Research designs are important because they are a way of protecting ourselves from ourselves!

True Experiments

The ideal study is designed as a true experiment. But even the best experiment needs to be replicated, hopefully by independent researchers. The reason for the lofty status of experiments is their ability to infer cause and effect relationships. The cause–effect connection is the result of a simple technique that makes comparison groups equal at the start of the experiment: *random assignment to groups*. If groups start out as equal, then the only possible explanation for different outcomes must be the result of different experimental conditions.

The Posttest-Only Control Group Design

The simplest and most familiar type of true experiment pits an experimental group against a control group when both have been created by random assignment:

$$R\text{-}X\text{-}O$$
$$R\qquad O$$

The imperfection in this study is in the blank space beneath the X. What was the control group actually doing while the experimental group was being examined? Imagine a marketing survey of a new film. A control group would be a more meaningful comparison group if they were watching a documentary of the same length as the film clip instead of wandering around a mall. This problem of random, uncontrolled influences on an experiment is usually referred to as *noise*.

The Pretest–Posttest Control Group Design

The critical feature of this design is random assignment to groups, and its importance is that it makes groups equal at the start of the experiment:

$$RO_1\text{-}X\text{-}O_2$$
$$RO_3\qquad O_4$$

Notice that symbolically, the R has replaced the dashes. Pay attention to the genius of random assignment to groups as you imagine testing the effectiveness of the 30-minute workshop in one hospital. The nurses are all different personalities; some drive long distances to get to work, and they will have different years of experience as nurses and at this particular hospital. Random assignment controls for all those factors (and more) by creating equivalence at the start of the experiment. The assignment to groups must be independent, random, and with enough participants to allow randomness to work its equalizing magic.

The effect of random assignment to groups is to place an equal mix of people in each group with diverse personalities, long commutes, years of service as a nurse, and every other individual difference that might systematically influence the scores on the Attitudes Towards Patients Scale. Here's what actually happens in this kind of a study:

Every participant completes the Attitudes Toward Patients Scale. A random half of the group then takes the 30-minute workshop while the other half engages in some different but equally engaging activity, such as completing a personality inventory.

Quasi-Experiments

Quasi-experimental designs are the practical landing place for many healthcare research projects. These almost-experimental designs acknowledge the importance of trying to control the thousands of confounding threats to clear scientific thinking. However, they recognize that there are many situations in which random assignment to groups is simply not possible, unethical, or pragmatically so expensive that important research questions will go neglected.

The Time-Series Design

The quasi-experimental time-series design looks like this:

$$O_1 O_2 O_3 O_4 X O_5 O_6 O_7 O_8$$

The time-series design reduces—but does not remove—one of the significant threats to clear scientific thinking: ignoring the surrounding *history* of your observation. For example, imagine that a college or university implemented a study skills workshop hoping that this exposure would increase students' private commitment to their education, measured by an EdCommitment Scale. A true experiment would use random assignment so that all students would experience the same campus environment, but one group of randomly selected students would participate in the workshop, and the other group would not.

However, several pragmatic forces (economics, staffing, local politics) make this sensible approach unlikely. In the absence of random assignment, the problem of history now threatens the logic of this study. For example, what if the campus were in turmoil over a controversial speaker, the firing of a popular professor, an outbreak of food poisoning, or simply enjoying spring break? A partial solution is to use a quasi-experimental time-series design that would measure educational commitment eight times so that any "bumps" from unanticipated historical events would be accounted for. This design has the added benefit of testing whether the effects of the workshop endure over time.

The Nonequivalent Control Group Design

The nonequivalent control group design looks like this:

O X O

O　　O

The idea of a quasi-experiment is to maximize control of alternative explanations when it is not possible to use random assignment to groups. The nonequivalent control group design is a commonly used approach that minimizes many threats to clear, scientific thinking. Long-time elementary school teachers seem to be especially sensitive to the value of this design. They tend to characterize each year's crop of students as distinct from one another using terms such as *bright*, *troublemakers*, *hardworking*, *unmotivated*, and *lazy*.

These two groups (above and below the dashed line) have not been formed through random assignment. Consequently, they are not equal, and their different starting points mean that we are interested in how much each group changes regardless of its raw scores. The usual hypothesis is that the group receiving the treatment (X) changed more than the other group.

Counterbalanced Designs

Within-groups experiments have a particular problem: *testing/order effects*. When every person in a study is exposed to every level of an experimental manipulation, experiencing one level may affect how they respond to the next level. For example, students who take the identical test two times in a row tend to perform better the second time around, especially if there has been a delay between the two tests (Leahy & Sweller, 2019). Why? Their working memories have been depleted immediately after the first test and enlarged by rumination or familiarity in the delayed condition. Whatever the cause, testing/order effects can be minimized (but not completely controlled) through a technique called *counterbalancing*, varying the order in which participants experience the experimental conditions. When there are three levels in this quasi-experimental design, the counterbalanced design creates six different orders of presentation and looks like this:

$$X_1O \quad X_2O \quad X_3O$$

$$X_1O \quad X_3O \quad X_2O$$

$$X_2O \quad X_1O \quad X_3O$$

$$X_2O \quad X_3O \quad X_1O$$

$$X_3O \quad X_1O \quad X_2O$$

$$X_3O \quad X_2O \quad X_1O$$

ROUNDUP

Human History in Six Sentences

The scientific principles of research design describe how humans have learned to think clearly. When confronted with diverse threats to their survival, our ancestors developed tools, weapons, and agriculture. We also learned to cooperate, live in groups, and create social systems that secured a better future for successive generations. With more successes than failures, our large brains slowly enabled us to think more clearly by accurately observing and interpreting the world around us. The guidelines for making trustworthy observations and interpretations gradually became formalized as scientific principles of research design. Over the last 500 years, those principles have gradually shifted the dominating influence on the human experience from superstition to science.

Connecting research designs to evolution is not a new idea. In a section subheaded with the words "Evolutionary Perspective on Cumulative Wisdom and Science," Donald Campbell and Julian Stanley (1966, p. 4) required only one sentence: "Experimentation … is a refining process superimposed upon the probably valuable cumulations of wise practice."

LINKS TO LEARN MORE

Introduction to research design: https://www.youtube.com/watch?v=GYyw R7SA03E

References

Campbell, D. T., & Stanley, J. C. (1966). *Experimental and quasi-experimental designs for research*. Chicago: R. McNally.

Dolan, R. J. (2007). Keynote address: Revaluing the orbital prefrontal cortex. *Annals of the New York Academy of Sciences, 1121*(1), 1–9. doi:10.1196/annals.1401.020

Feynman, R. P. (1974). Cargo cult science. *Caltech's 1974 commencement address.* Retrieved from http://calteches.library.caltech.edu/51/2/CargoCult.htm

Heinzen, T. E., & Goodfriend, W. (2019). *Case studies in social psychology: Critical thinking and application*. Thousand Oaks: SAGE.

Leahy, W., & Sweller, J. (2019). Cognitive load theory, resource depletion and the delayed testing effect. *Educational Psychology Review, 31,* 457–478. .doi:10.1007/s10648-019-09476-2

Macmillan, M. (2002). *An odd kind of fame: Stories of Phineas Gage.* Cambridge, MA: MIT Press.

Rolls, G. (2015). *Classic case studies in psychology.* London, UK: Routledge.

Toledo, A. H. (2004). The medical legacy of Benjamin Rush. *Journal of Investigative Surgery, 17*(2), 61–63. doi:10.1080/08941930490427785

Trivers, R. (2011). *The folly of fools: The logic of deceit and self-deception in human life.* New York, NY: Basic Books.

II

Starting the Actual Project

7

Qualitative, Quantitative, and Mixed Methods Research Designs

INTRODUCTION, or *First steps into considering data collection*

The method that you will engage to collect information (qualitative, quantitative, or mixed methods) to answer the research question will guide you as to the kind of data you need to collect and the strategies you will use for data analysis. Some questions will require numerical data that quantify the variables of interest, which can be obtained from surveys, systematic observations, and big data repositories. Other questions will require the development of a hypothesis or theory using exploratory methods through collecting information from focus groups, interviews, and observation/participation. The third method uses both of these approaches, with the subsequent outcomes offering additional support and depth in answering the question. This chapter is an introduction to these methods to assist the novice researcher in making a wise choice prior to embarking on a project.

Arriving at this juncture should be organic, starting from the identification of the discrepancy. It is the research question that evolves from the BIG PROBLEM, the discrepancy, the current problem, and the clarification of the aim/purpose that will direct you toward the best method to employ in your study.

OBJECTIVES

In this chapter you will learn:

- What is meant by quantitative research methods
- What constitutes qualitative research methods
- When to use a mixed methods approach
- How to clarify the question to help focus on the best method
- Ways to avoid the mousetraps that can undermine a good study

IMPORTANT DEFINITIONS

Some of the important vocabulary for this chapter includes the following:

Quantitative Research: This research method uses numerical data that can be analyzed through statistical inquiry. Quantitative research is structured in its approach. It can uncover patterns, reveal relationships, and be predictive in nature based on statistical probability. Sample size is very important in quantitative research to establish reliability and validity of outcomes.

Qualitative Research: This research method is exploratory by nature, providing the researcher with a deeper insight into a problem or event. Sample sizes are usually much smaller, but the information collected is richer in thoughts, opinions, and motivations.

Causality: Causality is an assumption that seeks to be established through rigorous research in some studies, demonstrating that the variable or factor that is being manipulated in the study (independent variable) is the reason for any change in the outcome (dependent variable). Establishing causality requires demonstrating relationships between the variables and meeting specific research conditions.

Probability: *Probability* is a statistical term that indicates likeliness of occurrence. It is used in sampling of a population and indicates that there is some level of randomness in which there is an equal possibility of each member of the sample being chosen.

Prospective: A prospective study is one that is happening in real time and moving forward in time with data collection.

Retrospective: A retrospective study looks to the past. It is one that examines data that have been collected in the past.

Correlation: A correlation is a relationship between two or more variables. It indicates that the variables are in some way related but not that one may be the cause of the other. A cardinal rule in research is that correlation does not mean causation.

WHERE DOES THE CHOICE OF RESEARCH METHODOLOGY FIT INTO THE RESEARCH PROCESS?

You may be sick of hearing this; however, it is imperative to understand that research is a total process, from problem to conclusion. It is like cultivating a flower; you have to identify the flower, examine the soil, find out what kind of food it needs, prepare the land, and then plant the seed, and then you are only halfway there! Choosing your method for research can be thought of as getting halfway toward the goal of finding some answers to better our understanding why there is a discrepancy in the big problem and maybe promote some possible ways to reduce the discrepancy (see Figure 7.1).

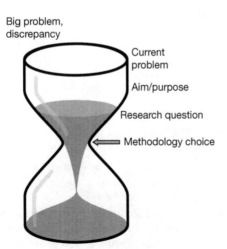

Figure 7.1 Hourglass of inquiry: The methodology choice.

QUANTITATIVE RESEARCH DESIGN BASICS

The four basic kinds of quantitative research designs are corre-lational designs, descriptive designs, experimental designs, and quasi-experimental designs. In all of these designs, the researcher is looking to identify if there is any correlation (relationship) between variables (factors of interest). These variables should be clarified in the aim/purpose and then specified in the research question. If the question that is being posed has to do with relationships that can be viewed by collecting numbers and comparing them, the methodology needed will be quantitative. When determining frequencies of an event or phenomenon is the study objective, frequency counts can be collected and analyzed. The questions being asked are as follows: *How much? How many?* The respondents in quantitative research usually provide replies on surveys and questionnaires, which ask closed-ended questions (*yes/no*, and Likert Scale responses with choices like *highly unlikely* to *highly likely*) that allow the researcher to quantify the answers. The answers are calibrated into scores and analyzed. Quantitative methods provide the ability for a researcher to get a broad breadth toward understanding a research problem by collecting data from large samples using questionnaires and surveys.

When calibrating scores, the researcher must be aware that all data are collected using a standardized method, to be certain that bias is not introduced that might affect the responses of the partici-pants. It is for this reason that quantitative research is seen as being somewhat distant, as the researcher does not want to engage the par-ticipant and alter an answer.

It is important to remember that quantitative research encom-passes identifying a limited number of variables (factors) to examine their relationships and interaction through the use of a large num-ber of cases. The types of variables used in quantitative research are dependent, independent, and controlled.

QUALITATIVE RESEARCH DESIGN BASICS

Qualitative research designs are focused on exploring, explain-ing, and developing deep understanding of specific phenomena. The kinds of questions that can be answered by qualitative research include these: *Why does...? How does...? What does it mean...?*

The questions are typically open-ended, which means that they require an explanation, not a yes/no or Likert-type sur-vey. Respondents in qualitative research can answer questions as they want, not directed by the researcher. Unlike the distant and nonengaging quantitative researcher's approach, the qualitative approach does not demand standardization of data and actually encourages researcher–participant interaction. Qualitative research allows the researcher to get a deeper understanding of a problem or phenomenon through interviews (structured and semistructured), analysis of images, and observations.

Qualitative research designs do not utilize variables as quantitative designs do. A qualitative design will not have the dependent and independent variable. The variable in qualitative research is called a categorical variable (fitting into a category) that can be described, but not quantified.

Fast Facts

Qualitative or Quantitative Method?
(answers at the end of the chapter)

1. A researcher wants to know how many students in ABC high school currently vape and if the number is increasing or decreasing. The school holds 1,500 students, all of whom take an anonymous survey at the start of each year, assessing substance use, including tobacco and vaping.
2. A researcher wants to know why some students choose to vape and others are smoking cigarettes.
3. A researcher wants to examine if there is a correlation between grade point average (GPA) of students who vape/smoke and those who do not.
4. A researcher wants to interview parents of students who smoke/vape and those who do not smoke/vape to learn their knowledge, attitudes, and own behaviors regarding smoking/vaping.
5. A researcher wants to survey students about their particular use of vaping paraphernalia and interview those who feel the need to carry their vaping case on them at all times.

MIXED METHODS RESEARCH DESIGN BASICS

Mixed methods has been identified as a third major research approach, also referred to as a research paradigm (Anguera, Blanco-Villaseñor, Losada, Sánchez-Algarra, & Onwuegbuzie, 2018; Johnson, Onwuegbuzie, & Turner, 2007). This approach utilizes data that are both qualitative and quantitative, wherein the evidence collected by

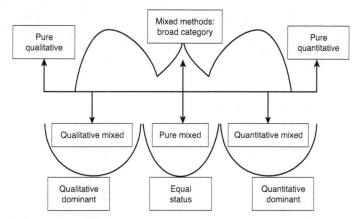

Figure 7.2 The mixed methods continuum.

Source: Adapted from Johnson, R. B, Onwuegbuzie, A. J., & Turner, L. A. (2007). Toward a definition of mixed methods research. *The Journal of Mixed Methods Research, 1*(2), 112–133. doi:10.1177/1558689806298224

the other methods deepens the understanding of the phenomenon being studied. Johnson et al. (2007) identify a mixed methods continuum, describing three types of mixed methods: qualitative dominant (qualitative mixed), equal status (pure mixed), and quantitative dominant (quantitative mixed), so named according to the amount of data that is derived from each subtype (see Figure 7.2).

Depending on the dominant research approach (qualitative or quantitative), the addition of the interview or survey provides a better understanding of the event or problem being scrutinized. The mixed methods approach usually works well for program evaluation, allowing the researcher to collect the standardized quantitative measurements for the program impact and then conducting interviews to determine individual experiences.

Tables 7.1 and 7.2 outline the process from Big Problem to study design for quantitative and qualitative or mixed methods design studies.

CHOOSING THE METHODOLOGY AND DESIGN THAT CAN BE A GOOD FIT FOR YOUR STUDY

If your study is looking to identify patterns of behaviors for populations or wants to collect information (either already collected, called archived data, or to be collected in real time) from questionnaires or surveys, you will probably be looking to engage in a study design that

Table 7.1

Setting Up the Quantitative Design Study From the Aim and Research Question

Big Problem	Aim/Purpose	Research Question	Quantitative Study Design
1. Vaping is a public health problem: adolescent vaping.	To determine if *the number* of students vaping is increasing each year.	Are students between the ages of 14 and 18 vaping in increasing numbers?	Utilizing the student risk-taking survey that is done at the start of each year, compare the number of student who say they vape over a period of 5 years.
2. Cigarette smoking is a public health problem.	To examine *other risk behaviors* of students who vape/smoke and those who do not for any correlation.	Is there a correlation between vaping/ smoking and engaging in other risky behaviors (drug use, truancy, risky sex)?	Utilizing the student risk-taking survey that is done each year, examine the variables of vaping/ smoking and other high-risk behaviors for correlations.

Table 7.2

Setting Up a Qualitative Design and Mixed Methods Design Study From the Aim and Research Question

Big Problem	Aim/Purpose	Research Question	Study Design
1. Vaping and smoking are a public health problem.	Identify *why some students choose* to vape and others are smoking cigarettes.	*Why do* some students vape and other smoke cigarettes?	Qualitative Study Design Interview three students who vape and three students who smoke to determine their reasons why.
2. Vaping is a public health problem.	Identify students' use of vaping paraphernalia, identifying those who feel the need to carry their vaping case on them at all times.	*How many* students feel the need to carry their vaping cases all the time, *and why* are they feeling that way?	Mixed Methods Study Design Implement a survey to identify students who state they need their vaping cases; then request interviews to determine reasons why.

will collect quantitative data. Quantitative data collection is focused on giving a breadth of information on a large number of people/subjects.

If, on the other hand, you are looking to get a deeper understanding of a phenomenon, to dive into the reasons why or the experiences of a phenomenon (either through looking at a historical period in depth or interviewing a person with a specific experience), you will probably be looking to engage in a study design that will utilize qualitative data. Qualitative data collection is focused on obtaining a depth of information from a few people/subjects.

Table 7.3 compares the two methods of data collection.

Now it is your turn. Before considering how to go about collecting your data, or even what data you need to collect, take some time to think about the problem, the aim, and the research question. See if you are able to fill in the information in the following Fast Facts box.

Fast Facts

Finding the method through clarifying the aim and the research question.

CURRENT PROBLEM: _____

DISCREPANCY: _____

BIG PROBLEM: _____

AIM/PURPOSE: _____

QUESTION: _____

Am I looking for objective patterns or statistical significance, or am I looking to get a deeper understanding of an idea or an experience?

METHOD OF DATA COLLECTION: _____

ROUNDUP

The aim/purpose and research question for a study will guide the researcher to identify what kind of data must be collected. Sometimes the question indicates actual numbers (how many, how much); other times the question is looking for levels of knowledge, attitudes, and beliefs (KAB) of a sample that can be determined through a questionnaire. When the answers to the questions can be quantified in a survey, the kind of data to be collected will be quantitative. When the questions indicate the desire to go deeper into feelings, experiences, or reasons why a person or event has occurred, the kind of

Table 7.3

Characteristics and Differences of Qualitative and Quantitative Research

Type of Research	Definition	Word Clues	Methods	Search Terms	Data	Researcher Role
Qualitative	"Investigations which use sensory methods such as listening or observing to gather and organize data into patterns or themes." (CINAHL)	• Ethnographic study • Field notes • Field research • Focus group • Observation • Open ended • Phenomenological	• Focus groups • Interviews • Recording behavior • Unstructured observation	• Qualitative studies (CINAHL) • Qualitative research (MEDLINE)	• Ideas • Interpretive • Narrative description • Text based • Words	Subjective: involved as a participant observer
Quantitative	"Scientific investigations in which numbers are used to measure variables such as characteristics, concepts, or things." (CINAHL)	• Case–control study • Lab experiment • Clinical trial • Cohort studies • Control group • Experimental group • Intervention • Randomized controlled trial • Statistical • Structured questionnaire	• Develops hypothesis • Determines methodology • Collects data • Analyzes data • Uses mathematical and statistical techniques to analyze data	• Quantitative studies (CINAHL) • MEDLINE uses headings for specific types of quantitative research; see the examples listed under Word Clues	• Measurable • Numbers • Statistics	Objective: separate, observes, but does not participate

CINAHL, Cumulative Index to Nursing and Allied Health Literature.

Source: Maricopa. (n.d.). *Qualitative versus quantitative research.* Retrieved from https://learn.maricopa.edu/courses/804760/pages/qualitative-versus-quantitative-research

Chapter 7 **Qualitative, Quantitative, and Mixed Methods Research Designs** data to answer that question will probably be qualitative. If a study wants to get information on a large group of people, but also wants to dive down into why some of those people are engaging in the event or behavior, a mixed methods approach will provide the needed answers. It is important to follow the aim/purpose of the study and to find the information that will answer the research question.

Answers to Fast Facts design questions on page 99: (1) quantitative—data mining from existing surveys, (2) qualitative, (3) quantitative, (4) qualitative, (5) mixed methods.

LINKS TO LEARN MORE

Qualitative vs. quantitative: https://www.youtube.com/watch?time_continue =10&v=2X-QSU6-hPU

References

Anguera, M. T., Blanco-Villaseñor, A., Losada, J. L., Sánchez-Algarra, P., & Onwuegbuzie, A. J. (2018, February). Revisiting the difference between mixed methods and multimethods: Is it all in the name? *Quality & Quantity, 52*(6), 2757–2770. doi:10.1007/s11135-018-0700-2

Johnson, R. B, Onwuegbuzie, A. J., & Turner, L. A. (2007). Toward a definition of mixed methods research. *The Journal of Mixed Methods Research, 1*(2), 112–133. doi:10.1177/1558689806298224

Maricopa. (n.d.). *Qualitative versus quantitative research.* Retrieved from https://learn.maricopa.edu/courses/804760/pages/qualitative-versus -quantitative-research

8

Methods of Data Collection

INTRODUCTION, or *How strong the bricks are will determine how strong the house will be*

The data, or information, you will be collecting will be the source of analysis in answering your research question. Once you have identified the Big Problem, discrepancy, current problem, aim, research question, and research design, it will be time to collect the data. The kind of data you will collect, the methods and tools you will use to collect the data, and the process you will use to store that data are all important in research. This chapter talks about choosing instruments to measure constructs (quantitative) as well as types of qualitative approaches to data collection. It also covers the importance of correct methods of data analysis and data storage.

OBJECTIVES

In this chapter you will learn:

- How the question and design guide the data
- About data collection processes
- About quantitative data collection
- How to identify methods to collect qualitative data
- What method of data collection would be best for your study

IMPORTANT DEFINITIONS

Some of the important vocabulary for this chapter includes the following:

Measurement Theory: Measurement theory examines the way we measure things. It uses a philosophical interpretation of the use of numerical measurements in research. Characteristics are assigned value that indicate a relationship to the characteristic (Fishburn, 2001).

Measurement Instruments: These instruments constitute the survey or other tool (e.g., interview questions) that a researcher will use to produce data for the study.

Operationalize: To operationalize means to identify the specific method to define and measure a variable. It allows the researcher to use surveys that quantify a construct or concept like attitude.

Self-Report Data: This information is provided to the researcher by the subject, either through a survey or through an interview process.

Open-Ended Questions: These questions require an explanation as an answer. Usually open-ended questions begin with the words *how, why, when, where,* and *what.*

Closed-Ended Questions: These questions can be answered by a simple yes, no, or maybe, or can be quantified on a survey with a Likert-scaled response.

Likert-Type Scale: Named after Rensis Likert, this scale quantifies answers on a survey that rates a person's attitude, value, or opinion on a topic. Sometimes the scale is more broadly referred to as a rating scale.

Trustworthiness: This term reflects the level of credibility and objectivity found in the results of a research project. It is usually based upon a number of qualities like transferability, dependability, and confirmability. Validity and reliability are very important in establishing trustworthiness.

Precision: The precision of an instrument can also be considered the reliability measure. Establishing precision in evaluation requires that there is demonstrated accuracy in the tool.

MEASUREMENT PRINCIPLES AND DATA COLLECTION

The quality of a house you might build will depend upon the quality of the materials you use to construct it. You might have chosen the perfect neighborhood, hired the best architect, and have the picture-perfect blueprint, but if you do not use quality building components, your house may not be strong enough to withstand the first storm. A research study, just like a home, needs to be built with tested, precise, accurate, and trustworthy measures.

The measurement theory examines the way we measure things, the kinds of things we can actually measure, the relationship between measures, and how errors can be made during the measurement process (Allen & Yen, 2001). This is important because many of the measures that are collected in research *represent* a construct, which is not usually a number with a true value. For example, a survey may ask questions about likes and dislikes, assigning numbers from 1 to 5 with 1 meaning "do not like at all" and 5 meaning "like a lot." Those numbers have been given meaning by the questionnaire, how much a person likes something, but the numbers themselves do not measure anything, and the assigning of numbers is simply a way for the researcher to measure an emotion (like). The research question reflects the aim of the study and identifies the variables of interest to be studied. These variables will need to be defined in measurable components in order to be analyzed and interpreted. This is called operationalizing a construct by using a scale or a questionnaire.

Fast Facts

Linking the Current Known Elements of a Research Study to Data Collection

It is a fact that there are data collection methods that are better fits depending on the research approach. Qualitative, quantitative, and mixed methods approaches may employ different data collection methods in order to arrive at results that can clarify, deepen understanding of, or predict an event, phenomenon, or behavior.

The design of the study is the first indicator: If the study is looking at a causal or relationship phenomenon, data collection will need to have a certain level of preciseness and control (Norwood, 2010). The quantitative and mixed methods approaches will require some level of controlling variables in the research situation. If, on the other hand, the approach is purely qualitative, the data collection method will not seek to control variables, nor to collect information from large unknown samples.

MEASUREMENT INSTRUMENTS

Quantitative Measurement Instruments

Research that uses a quantitative design will be collecting information that either exists in numerical form or can be translated into numbers for evaluation. The tool or instrument that the researcher will use must accurately measure the variables under question. Accuracy is reflected in the reliability and validity of the instrument, concepts that are examined more closely in Chapter 9, "Reliability and Validity." Using instruments that lack reliability and validity will provide outcomes that are not considered believable. Most existing tools are evaluated for their reliability and validity, with these characteristics reported in the psychometrics (or tested measures) of the instrument.

There are two ways to measure the variables: either directly or indirectly. Types of instruments for quantitative design studies include questionnaires, document analysis instruments, medical reports, and direct, quantifiable observations.

Direct Measures

The direct measure provides exact, concrete information about the factor of interest and does not need to be interpreted in any other way. These variables are represented in tangible characteristics like height, weight, age, and body temperature. Each of these characteristics has scales, or measurement tools, that can provide the data needed. A researcher who wants to look at the body heaviness of athletes, for example, might use a weight scale as the measuring instrument and get a direct reading of the person's weight. If, on the other hand, the researcher was interested in a student's understanding of research methods, a test or exam might be the tool to use. It is important to keep in mind that a direct measure needs no other interpretation as it provides specific information related to your factors.

Indirect Measures

Indirect measures are less concrete than direct measures. These measures might reflect attitudes, perceptions, feelings, or beliefs of a person, and usually they are collected through the use of self-report instruments. Rather than stating the fact, indirect measures imply the construct of interest when the variable is not able to be seen directly, like values, beliefs, and attitudes. The measurement tools used to collect indirect measures are usually surveys, interviews, reports, and evaluations. A researcher who wants to know the impact of a teacher's teaching style on students' learning might employ an evaluation by the students. The students would fill out the survey (self-report), highlighting what they feel about the teacher's style on their learning.

Fast Facts

Direct or Indirect?
Answers at the end of the chapter

What kind of measures are being collected below: direct or indirect?

1. A researcher wants to know the blood glucose level of people with A1C levels of 3.5.
2. A school wants to evaluate the impact of an 11 p.m. curfew on the sense of safety in the community.
3. Pat fills out a survey related to the likelihood of returning for another meal in a particular restaurant.
4. The police are evaluating the effect of reducing the speed limit on pedestrian strikes.
5. The weather person is examining rainfall totals during a month's period and comparing it to the rainfall totals in the same month a year ago.

Qualitative Measurement Instruments

Qualitative research is investigation that can generate new theories, provide a deeper understanding of a phenomenon, and present a level of detail not usually represented in quantitative studies. Qualitative studies examine content and themes, and most importantly, the instrument used to collect the data is the researcher. The outcome of qualitative research is reflected in a narrative. This is not to say that the construct of interest is not examined; it is just that the data are collected by the researcher and also examined by the researcher to identify themes and patterns providing insight into the concept of interest.

QUANTITATIVE MEASUREMENT

Levels of Measurement in Quantitative Research

There are four measurement levels (scales) in quantitative research: nominal, ordinal, interval, and ratio.

Nominal Scale

A nominal scale is one that attaches an arbitrary number to a category or name; that number has no value *except* that it indicates the category or name. This number is actually representing qualities, not quantities of a variable. An example of this is attaching a number to represent a person's sex: 1 = male, 2 = female, 3 = transgender, and so on. The numbers 1, 2, and 3 have no actual importance in magnitude, only that they represent an answer that can be grouped at a later time to investigate characteristics of the subjects. A higher number is not more valuable. It does not provide any qualifications on the data; it simply represents a category of something. An important fact to consider when assigning characteristics to a nominal scale is to provide the respondents with enough choices so that they will respond. This is a closed-ended question, so the subject *must* choose from the answers provided. If only one answer can be chosen by the respondent, be certain to group the categories so that they are mutually exclusive; a person should not be able to fit into two categories (Wood & Ross-Kerr, 2011). The researcher, before identifying nominal data for collection, must consider all the possible responses that might fit into a given category, including *prefer not to answer* or *other*.

The purpose of nominal data is to allow the researcher to count (quantify) how many respondents or subjects belong to a specific characteristic or category.

Examples of nominal categories: presence of illness symptoms (e.g., cough, fever, chest pain), gender (e.g., M, F, T, other), sexual orientation (e.g., L, G, B, Q, other), academic major (e.g., nursing, public health, communication disorders), school attended, purpose of visit to an urgi-center (e.g., wellness check, cold/flu, prescription renewal).

Fast Facts

Limitations of Nominal Data

A limitation of nominal data is that it simply provides a concrete answer to a question, where the respondent has one choice and must fit into the characteristic(s) identified by the researcher. One clear example of this is race, where the response may not be clearly one race or another, and biracial might not be expressive or informational enough. Can you think of others?

Ordinal Scale

An ordinal scale is one in which the number has some meaning, but that meaning is not absolute. This scale places responses related to a category in a specific order indicating either increasing or decreasing magnitude. The ordinal scale ranks the characteristic, rather than just placing it in a category with an arbitrary number. If something is ranked from 1 to 4, those in category 4 are at a greater magnitude of the characteristic than those at level 1. Unlike nominal data, the numbers in ordinal data do have a meaning; the higher the number, the greater the presence of the characteristic. Unfortunately, the kind of information a researcher can get from ordinal data is very limited. Although it ranks the characteristic, it does not provide exact information.

The purpose of collecting ordinal data is to provide a ranking of categories or characteristics of a sample. The number assigned indicates rank only, not specific quantified characteristics.

Examples of ordinal data: level of education (e.g., freshman = 1, sophomore = 2, junior = 3, senior = 4), age group (e.g., child = 1, adolescent = 2, young adult = 3, adult = 4, senior citizen = 5).

Fast Facts

Limitations of Ordinal Data

Information collected by using ordinal data also has limitations that the researcher should be aware of prior to the collection of information from the respondent. Because ordinal scales form categories of characteristics, it is the researcher who will be defining these categories and ordering them. They do not give the actual quantified level of expertise, skill, or characteristic that is being measured, but rather a sliding kind of scale. A good example of this, which many students dislike, is the use of categories A through D for grading, in which a student with an A average might actually have a 100 on all the tests or maybe only a 91, but both would be grouped as an A. Age is often described as an ordinal number, which presents the problem during analysis if the groupings are so large that they do not provide the information needed.

Where possible, researchers should seek interval and ratio data. Can you think of other kinds of ordinal data that impose limitations on the analysis?

Interval Scale and Ratio Scale

The interval and ratio scales, distinguished from the previous two scales (nominal and ordinal), are considered quantitative numeric scales in which the numbers have a real meaning.

Interval Data. The numbers in an interval scale are indicative of real quantifiable characteristics, represented by numbers that have equal distances between them. They have both order (higher numbers are greater magnitude) and exact value. For example, temperatures are considered interval data. The one degree between temperatures is always the same; the same distance between 98° and 99° is equal to the distance between 100° and 101°. These numbers represent the level of warmth by providing a numerical temperature. What is important to consider is that if the temperature is 0, that 0 does not mean that there is no temperature. Zero usually is an indication that something does not exist. If I have 0 apples, I have no apples, but if it is 0° outside, there is still a temperature. So in interval data the number 0 is not an absolute, just another number on the scale.

The purpose of interval data is to report characteristics that can be measured and have equidistance to each other on established continuums, where the number 0 is just another number, not indicative of the absence of the characteristic.

Examples of interval data: temperature (Celsius and Fahrenheit), time as measured on a 24-hour clock. Can you think of others?

Ratio Data. This scale is like the interval data scale with two important differences. A 0 in ratio data has a real meaning, indicating the characteristic being measured is absent and there are no negative numbers in ratio data. Once there is nothing left (0), there is nothing to count. When a researcher is considering whether the data are interval or ratio, it is important to determine if a reading of 0 reflects just another point on a continuum or if it is an absolute number that tells the researcher something does not exist.

The purpose of ratio data is to allow the researcher to calculate the quantitative existence of a variable of interest and report trends in relationships using specific statistical methods of analysis.

Examples of ratio data: a person's weight, number of children, age, height, blood count, pulse, blood pressure, tire pressure. Can you think of others?

Methods to Collect Quantitative Data

If a researcher is going to collect data and assign numerical values to the data, it will be considered quantitative data collection. The methods might include the examination of demographics (characteristics about your respondents) and specific attributes or variables that are quantified using nominal, ordinal, interval, and ratio data. Methods that can be employed to collect this kind of data are surveys, questionnaires, observations, reports, and data mining.

QUALITATIVE MEASUREMENT

Levels of Measurement in Qualitative Research

Just as in quantitative research, the qualities of interest in qualitative studies need to be categorized for analysis in order to arrive at their narrative. Though the phenomenon being investigated might be grouped in categories and some may be assigned a numerical code, the majority of the qualitative measures will employ nominal and/ or ordinal data, facilitating the coding of groups for analysis. All levels of measurement can be collected for qualitative research that will reflect some of the variables under investigation. An example of this is asking the age of the participants and indicating that number in the results. The analysis of the data, however, in a qualitative research study will be focused on the deeper investigation that can produce an deep understanding of an event or phenomenon that occurs in the natural setting. The small samples used in qualitative research underscore the importance of the narrative rather than the quantifiable comparisons and relationships between variables in large samples. It is important to remember a qualitative study could have a sample size as small as 1 (case study); the definitive attribute in the qualitative approach is the depth of investigation, not the breadth.

The kinds of nominal data that could be collected for qualitative research (studies that explore experiences, events, people, and cultures using small samples but gathering deep data) might include a person's belief on death associated with his or her religion or the affiliation with a specific political party. The types of ordinal level measurements might be pain levels or movie ratings (from G to X), with the meaning of the numbers ranking the movies associated with deeper feelings that can be investigated by the researcher.

Methods to Collect Qualitative Data

Surveys are often employed at the outset of a qualitative research study to identify participants; however, because the sample numbers are usually smaller in qualitative research, and the level of investigation seeks to go deeply into the phenomenon, personal interviews, focused observations, and use of archival data (content analysis) are the most common methods used to collect qualitative data.

WHAT DATA COLLECTION METHOD IS BEST FOR YOUR STUDY?

This is where you must, once again, go back to the hourglass of your study (Figure 8.1). It is time to determine how exactly you will measure the answer to the question.

If your question reflects an aim of testing a hypothesis that includes a cause-and-effect scenario or is attempting to predict a behavior or occurrence (e.g., health providers' attitudes related to medicating foreign-born women during childbirth) or describe a trend in a population (e.g., use of pain medications on young non-English-speaking immigrant women during childbirth), you are leaning toward a quantitative method of data collection. In this instance you might use randomly selected healthcare providers and conduct a survey identifying attitudes and behaviors, using numbers and statistics to identify if a statistical relationship exists between attitudes of healthcare providers toward immigrant women and likelihood of providing pain medication during childbirth. You will not know your participants in the study, and your subjects will not know your beliefs or biases.

The research question starts with *How many..., How much..., How often..., How regularly..., What are the differences (similarities)...,* or *What is the relationship between...?* Can you think of other beginnings to quantitative research questions?

If, however, the aim of your study is to get an understanding of and interpretation of an identified phenomenon (pain treatment of childbirth) using an intentionally small specific sample (young

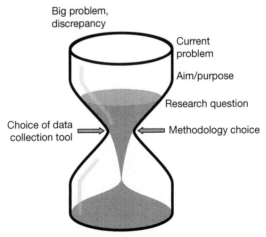

Figure 8.1   Hourglass of inquiry: Choosing a data collection tool.

non-Anglophone immigrant females), which will increase the understanding of the childbirth experience of the subject(s), then you would be more likely to use a qualitative method to collect your information. This might include open-ended interviews, observations, and focus groups. In this case you would be looking to uncover patterns, themes, and other features that are uncovered during the interviews. In this research, you may get to know your participants, and your relationship with those participants can be included as part of your study. Qualitative research questions often start with a *what, does, how,* and *why*. Some qualitative research questions might be *What are the lived experiences of...? Does anxiety impact empathy in...? How does breastfeeding change early motherhood...?* and *Why do some grandchildren of Holocaust survivors exhibit symptoms of posttraumatic stress disorder (PTSD)?*

See if you are able to fill in the information in the following Fast Facts box.

Fast Facts

Identifying a Data Collection Method

AIM/PURPOSE: _____

QUESTION: _____

Am I interested in identifying patterns, using larger samples, and predicting trends? Y ___ N ___

Am I interested in looking at a small group of people and examining a specific experienced phenomenon with the aim of describing it in depth? Y ___ N ___

VARIABLE(S) OF INTEREST: _____

METHOD TO COLLECT INFORMATION THAT CAN ANSWER MY QUESTION: _____

ROUNDUP

Constructing a clear research question that grows out of the problem, discrepancy, and aim of the study assists the researcher in identifying the kind of research method to use, which in turn clarifies what kind of instrument or approach will yield the desired data. Understanding the types of data—nominal, ordinal, interval, and ratio—and their strengths and limitations in providing answers is an important factor to be considered before starting the data collection process. Some novice researchers might consider making up their own surveys, which can be problematic to the validity of the research results. The literature search can identify existing surveys that have been tested and found to be reliable and valid and should be the novice researchers' first choice when collecting data. Chapter 9, "Reliability and Validity," explores the importance of valid and reliable research tools as well as the trustworthiness aspect of qualitative designs.

ANSWERS TO FAST FACTS: DIRECT OR INDIRECT

1. direct; 2. indirect; 3. indirect; 4. direct; 5. direct

LINKS TO LEARN MORE

Qualitative vs. quantitative: https://www.youtube.com/watch?v=2X-QSU6-hPU

Quantitative vs. qualitative data: https://www.youtube.com/watch?v=EcKrT_IegoU

References

Allen, M. J., & Yen, W. M. (2001). *Introduction to measurement theory*. Long Grove, IL: Waveland Press.

Fishburn, P. (2001). Measurement theory. In N. J. Swelser & P. B. Baltes (Eds.), *International Encyclopedia of the Social and Behavioral Sciences* (pp. 9448–9451). Retrieved from https://www.sciencedirect.com/topics/chemical-engineering/measurement-theory

Norwood, S. L. (2010). *Research essentials: Foundations for evidence based practice*. Upper Saddle River, NJ: Pearson Education.

Wood, M. J, & Ross-Kerr, J. C. (2011). *Basic steps in planning nursing research: From question to proposal* (7th ed.). Sudbury, MA: Jones & Bartlett.

9

Reliability and Validity

Katherine Roberts

INTRODUCTION, or *Who cares if it is reliable or valid?*

This chapter focuses on the basic principles of reliability and validity and the importance of establishing trustworthiness of your data. Without reliability and validity, the data you collect will not be able to provide answers to your research questions. Establishing reliability and validity is essential regardless if you are collecting qualitative or quantitative data.

OBJECTIVES

In this chapter you will learn:

- The importance of reliability
- How to measure reliability of your data
- Ways to establish construct validity
- Multiple methods of assessing validity
- Why it is necessary to establish both reliability and validity

IMPORTANT DEFINITIONS

Some of the important vocabulary for this chapter includes the following:

Reliability: Reliability is the extent to which data are consistent.

Validity: Validity is the extent to which the instrument measures the construct that it is supposed to measure.

Concept: A concept identifies an abstract object or phenomenon and is often used to present an idea that is connected to a theory.

Construct: Constructs may include multiple concepts. They cannot be directly measured but can be inferred through measurable variables, like behaviors.

Operational Definition: This statement of what is going to be studied and how it will be measured is specifically related to your concepts and conceptual/theoretical framework, if you have identified one for your study.

ESTABLISHING RELIABILITY AND VALIDITY

Establishing reliability and validity related to your measurement tools and data collected about the variables is of utmost importance to your research study. It is also crucial to examine when evaluating the research reports of others. After all, how likely are you to trust what you read if the results are not valid and the outcomes are not reliable? When we collect data and then report on the results of data we collect, we need to ask similar questions as we did in Chapter 1, "Introduction to Research," only this time, we are focusing on the data. We ask:

- How do I know that I can believe these data?
- How can I trust the results of these data?

Imagine that you just purchased an electric scooter to take you to the beach. The first day you get on the scooter, and it takes you exactly 5 minutes to go the 1 mile to the beach. You do this for 8 days straight, and each time it takes you 5 minutes, so you assume, if nothing changes, the time spent on your scooter is considered a reliable measure of distance. If you get on your scooter for 10 minutes, that means you have covered a distance of 2 miles. However, one day there is bad weather, and the roads are wet. And it takes you over 6 minutes to get to the beach. Does that mean you went farther than a mile that day? No, it means that the variable of weather resulted in measurement error and made the data you collected less accurate. There was inconsistency in the data you collected.

Reliability refers to the consistency or stability of your data. Reliable data contain little measurement error, meaning these data are accurate. If you collected data on the distance to the beach with your GPS fitness app, you will get the same results every time regardless of the weather, so these data would be considered reliable. If you collect data on the distance to the beach by how long it takes you on your scooter, you may get different results from day to day; therefore, there is a lot of measurement error using time on your scooter to measure distance.

Classical test theory states that there will always be some error in measurement.

Observed Score (O) = True Score (T) + Error Score (E)

O = observed score: the values or the scores we have obtained with our measurement instrument

T = true score: the score that would have been obtained if our measurement instrument was free from all errors

E = error score: measurement error

Fast Facts

Random Versus Systematic Error

Joe came for a blood pressure (BP) reading. The nurse took his BP, and it was 150/90. When she tells Joe this, he says "Great! It's usually much higher!" The nurse takes his pressure on the other arm, waits a few minutes, and repeats it. The resulting readings were 160/90, 156/86, and 150/90.

It is well known that BP, on the same person, can fluctuate across readings. This is due to *random error*. In order to reduce error and obtain a more accurate measure of the patient's actual BP, several readings can be taken and averaged together.

If Joe, on the other hand, tells the nurse that he normally has a BP of 120/70, but sometimes when it is tested in the doctor's office it reads much higher, this reading might be reflective of a systematic error because of Joe's particular characteristic of experiencing white coat syndrome.

A person might experience high stress or anxiety when the person get his or her BP measured at a hospital or doctor's office (white coat syndrome). The white coat syndrome can result in a consistently elevated BP reading in those environments. Taking multiple readings and getting an average would not eliminate this error. This reading would be considered inaccurate because of *systematic error*.

Error can be either *random error* (affects the score because of purely chance happenings) or *systematic error* (affects the scores because of some particular characteristic of the person or the test that has nothing to do with the construct being measured; Crocker & Algina, 1986).

RELIABILITY OF A MEASUREMENT TOOL

A measure needs to be constructed in a way that data collected from it is consistent and stable. This can get a little tricky. Although we talk about how measures are reliable, in reality, reliability is a function of data, not instrumentation (Nimon, Zientek, & Henson, 2012). For example, you can use a measurement instrument (like a survey) that has produced reliable data in the past. However, when *you* use this measurement instrument, your study sample may have different characteristics than the original sample, or there may be more systematic error during your data collection process. Owing to these possibilities, the data you collect may not be as reliable, even though you used the same exact measurement instrument. Therefore, it is important that researchers assess the reliability of their data and not just reference the reliability statistic from prior research, assuming that the same level of reliability applies to their data. If the data we collect are not reliable, then the conclusions we draw on the basis of such data may not be correct. The results may not be able to be replicated and, therefore, will not be believable.

Most methods for estimating reliability produce a number called a reliability coefficient (or a coefficient of stability), which is a correlation coefficient that ranges in value from 0.0 to 1.0. In data with perfect reliability, the reliability coefficient is 1.0, and there would be no error. On the other hand, when the reliability coefficient is 0.0, this means that all variability is due to measurement error and none is coming from the true score. Coefficients at or above 0.80 are often considered sufficiently reliable to make decisions about individuals based on their observed scores (Webb, Shavelson, & Haertel, 2006). Lower reliability may be acceptable in new areas of research or theory testing, and high reliability is critical for diagnostic testing (e.g., clinical depression, weight) or predictive studies. However, note that reliability should not be the only consideration in decisions about the appropriateness of test uses or interpretations.

How Do We Assess Reliability?

Reliability cannot be directly known because that would require one to know the true score, which, according to classical test theory, is not possible because there is always error. But it is very important that we know approximate reliability. Fortunately estimates of reliability can be obtained by various means (many of which you might already know), including test–retest, parallel-form, interrater, and internal consistency.

Test-Retest Reliability

Test–retest reliability establishes consistency of a measure across time. To assess this type of reliability, a measurement instrument is administered to the same subjects at two different points in time.

Test = time one
Retest = time two (usually around 7–20 days)

The researcher then looks for a relationship (correlation) between the results of the two administrations. Ideally, you want to see a high correlation coefficient, which would indicate no substantial change between the two results. This indicates that the data reflect the true score with low measurement error. Some *drawbacks* to conducting this type of reliability is that subjects may remember how they responded on the first test, so the correlation could be falsely high. Or alternatively, the correlation could be low because the subjects may have more error at first administration owing to being unfamiliar with the test compared to the later administration. If you collect baseline data and then the results change a week later without doing anything, the data are not sufficiently reliable to assess change over time due to your intervention/program.

Parallel-form Reliability

To assess parallel-form reliability, subjects take two different forms of a measurement instrument at the same time, and then the results are correlated to see how consistent they are with each other. If both forms reflect the meaning of the complex idea that is being tested (capture the domain of the construct), they should be highly correlated, and therefore, either one is reliable. The advantage of this type of reliability over test–retest reliability is that there is no time between measures; it will be done all in one sitting. *Disadvantage:* It is quite challenging to make parallel forms of an instrument. You can create a large set of questions and then randomly divide the questions to create the two forms, but this is difficult, and by chance, you may not get equivalent tests. If you end up with equivalent forms, however, you can use one as a pretest and one as a posttest, eliminating the possibility that subjects might remember questions from the pretest, which could confound results.

Interrater Reliability

Establishing consistency with this type of reliability means the researcher is looking for consistency across raters or observers. To assess interrater reliability, two or more raters are required to score the same set of subjects or information, after which their results are compared. If there is consistency across the raters in their scoring, you have established high interrater reliability. If raters are used in your study, this reliability is important to assess at the beginning of a study to ensure there is consistency, but it is also important to assess them from time to time during the study to make sure that the raters are not drifting apart in their scoring.

Internal Consistency Reliability

Determining dependability of results with this type of reliability means looking for consistency across items on a multiple-item instrument. Generally, items on a scale or an instrument are supposed to reflect the same underlying construct, so the scores on those items should be correlated with each other. To assess internal consistency, the correlation between the individual items and total score is examined. If reliability is high, then it suggests that the items are measuring the same construct, and therefore, there is internal consistency within the set of items. Measures of internal consistency are the most commonly reported form of reliability coefficient because they are readily available from a single administration of a test. There is no need to repeat an administration of a measure as would be needed in test–retest, and there is no need for a different instrument as in parallel forms.

Fast Facts

Reliability of a Step Counter

Pat got a step counter from Sheri, a good friend, who assured Pat of the reliability of the counter. She told Pat that the number of steps between their homes was 6,000.

When Pat used the counter, the number of steps registered 4,700. What could have impacted the number of steps? Was it a problem with the measurement tool (step counter)?

Pat has much longer legs than Sheri. So although the counter indicated 6,000 steps for Sheri, it only registered 4,700 for Pat. The counter needed to be recalibrated for Pat.

(continued)

(continued)

Remember that even if you have a measure that in the past has been shown to produce reliable data, that does not mean when you use that measure, the data you collect will automatically be reliable. However, using a measure that has been shown to produce reliable data in the past can reduce the likelihood that you will have unreliable data.

VALIDITY

Remember that scooter from the beginning of the chapter? Let's go back to it. The first time you have to travel to the beach on your electric scooter, you are given a map. You know you will go 1 mile in 10 minutes. But, does the map actually take you there? How believable is that map? What if that map was made in the 1800s—back then it was thought to be valid. But, today, the landscape has changed with additional roads and beach erosion, so what we thought we were measuring (distance to the beach) is not actually what we are measuring with this old map.

Validity is the extent to which the instrument measures what it purports to measure. *You cannot have validity if your data are not reliable*; because there will be so much inconsistency in your data, it will provide no meaningful interpretation. However, *you can have reliability without validity* if the data are consistent but these findings do not represent what you intended to measure. In the ideal situation you have both reliability and validity (Figure 9.1).

Fast Facts

Validity of a Weight Scale

Pat and Sheri work out together, and Sheri, who wears a size 12, decides to step on the scale at the gym. Pat, who is taller than Sheri and wears a size 6, lets Sheri know that she had been to the doctor that morning and she knows her current weight to be 120 lb.

Sheri gets on the scale, which reads 120 lb, a 15-lb loss from the weight she was told at her doctor's office 2 weeks before. She gets off the scale and gets back on, and low and behold, the scale reads 120 lb again. "See," she says to Pat, "this is a very reliable scale!" Pat then gets on the scale, and it reads the same as Sheri at 120 lb. Sheri tells Pat that she must have really lost 15 lb!

(continued)

(continued)

A trainer comes in and sees the women on the scale. "Come with me" she tells the women and leads them into the private gym, which has a medical standard upright scale. Pat gets on the scale, and it reads 120 lb; then Sheri gets on the scale, and it reads 135 lb, the same weight she had been told at her doctor's office weeks before. The women reweighed themselves on the standup scale two more times, receiving the same weights each time.

The first scale was reliable in that it provided the same reading time and again, but unfortunately it was not a valid reading. A scale can be reliable without being valid.

The second scale provided a valid weight, which was also reliable. A valid measurement tool must also be reliable.

ROBIN HOOD SCENARIO

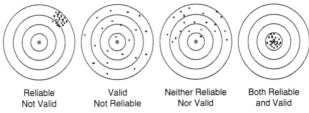

Reliable   Valid   Neither Reliable   Both Reliable
Not Valid   Not Reliable   Nor Valid   and Valid

Figure 9.1 Robin Hood scenario of reliability and validity.

Source: From Trochim, W. M. K., Donnelly, J. P., & Arora, K. (2016). *The research methods: The essential knowledge base* (2nd ed.). Boston, MA: Cengage Learning. Reproduced by permission.

The preceding figure (Figure 9.1) shows four possible scenarios.

■ In the first scenario, you are hitting the target consistently, but you are missing the center of the target. That is, you are consistently and systematically measuring the wrong value. This measure is reliable, but not valid (i.e., it is consistent but wrong).

■ In the second scenario, you are randomly hitting the target. You seldom hit the center of the target, but if you take the average of all your hits, you are getting the right answer for the group (but not very well for individuals). In this case, you get a valid group estimate, but you are inconsistent.

- The third scenario shows that your hits are spread across the target and you are consistently missing the center. Your measure in this case is neither reliable nor valid.
- In the fourth scenario, which is the "Robin Hood" scenario, you are consistently hitting the center of the target. Your measure is both reliable and valid.

Construct Validity

A construct, as you will remember, is a complex idea that we try to measure in research. So, when we examine construct validity, we are interested in identifying whether the instrument we are using actually measures the construct it claims to be measuring. Many constructs cannot be measured directly. This is because, as complex ideas, they are usually hypothetical in nature, so the researcher must first develop the conceptual definitions reflecting the constructs. This conceptual definition is then transformed by the measurement tool into an operational definition.

Creating the Operational Definition

To create an operational definition, we need to both clearly define the concept and state how we will measure it. For example, we cannot directly measure the construct of depression, so we need to operationally define what depression is, such as feeling sad. Then we need to decide how we will measure this construct. We can use a measure that already has strong evidence of validity, such as the Center for Epidemiologic Studies Depression Scale Revised (cesd-r.com; Van Dam & Earleywine, 2011), which asks questions about feeling depressed, feeling hopeful, feeling lonely, and so on. Although we cannot be sure that this instrument completely measures the construct of depression, this measure has undergone multiple different methods to establish its validity, and those tests have been published in peer-reviewed journals. The existence of evidence on the validity of this tool allows us to determine that this measure is a valid representation of the hypothetical construct of depression.

Indicators of Construct Validity

Face Validity

Does the instrument, on the face of it, appear to measure what it claims to measure? Face validity is subjective in that it relies on judgment. Although it is the easiest form of validity to apply, it is thought to be the weakest indicator of validity. In order to determine if a measure has face validity, you read through the questions and ask yourself if they appear to be an accurate operational definition of the construct. To improve the quality of face validity, you can show it to experts and get their opinion on whether the instrument has face validity. However, realize that appearance is not a very good indicator of validity.

Content Validity

Is the content of the instrument representative of the entire domain of a given construct? This type of validity examines if the items developed to operationalize a construct provide an adequate and representative sample of all the items that might measure the construct. Similar to face validity, content validity usually depends on judgment of experts in the field to determine if the measure adequately covers a content area or adequately represents a construct.

Criterion-Related Validity

How well does the instrument compare with an external criterion, such as an acceptable measure? This type of validity examines how scores on an instrument correlate with other measures of the same construct or similar underlying constructs that are theoretically related. Four common types of criterion-related validity are predictive validity, concurrent validity, convergent validity, and discriminant validity.

Predictive Validity Do scores on the instrument *predict* behavior or performance on a criterion measured at a future time? At the time of the administration of the measure, this criterion or future behavior is unknown. The criterion measurement is obtained at some time after the administration of the instrument, and then it is determined if the measure accurately predicts the criterion. For example, after conducting decades-long follow-up studies, evidence suggested that blood pressure is a predictable risk factor for cardiovascular disease. A major drawback for testing for predictive validity is that it can be costly and time intensive.

Concurrent Validity Are scores on an instrument related to scores from a criterion measure of the same construct administered *concurrently* in the same subjects? This type of validity is common when developing a new measure to take the place of the gold standard measure of the construct. The new measure may have some advantage over the gold standard measure, such as being shorter and less time-consuming to complete. For example, a single-item measure for depression among cardiac inpatients, which required no additional scoring and was free of charge, was compared with another previously validated measure of depression and was found to have high concurrent validity (Young, Nguyen, Roth, Broadberry, & Mackay, 2015).

Convergent Validity Are scores on an instrument similar or related to scores on another that measures the same construct? Similar to the word *converge*, which is defined as "to come together and unite in a common interest or focus" ("Converge," n.d.), when you have convergent validity, your measure is highly correlated to those of the same construct or similar construct.

Divergent Validity This is the opposite of convergent validity; in divergent validity the scores on an instrument should not be similar to those that are actually unrelated, meaning that the instrument should not be highly correlated with other tests designed to measure theoretically different concepts. If it is not divergent enough, then maybe you are actually not measuring what you think you are measuring, or it suggests that the tests are measuring the same thing and are too alike to be considered different. For example, Wallach and Kogan's (1965) classic study of 151 children demonstrated that tests of creativity did not correlate with tests of intelligence and academic achievement (average $r = .09$). Therefore, these tests were measuring different constructs.

Fast Facts

Keys to Selecting a Valid and Reliable Instrument to Use

- Look for evidence of reliability and validity by conducting a literature search on the instrument.
- Review prior studies that have reported validity and reliability.
- Examine the purpose for which the instrument was used.
- Examine the sample and setting in which the instrument was used.
- Determine if the instrument has been used in a population and setting similar to the one you will be studying.
- Determine if estimates of reliability are high and have been obtained through multiple methods.
- Evaluate the evidence provided that the measure is a valid representative of the construct.

ROUNDUP

The reliability and validity of the measurement tools chosen to measure the variables and constructs in a study are of major importance. It is the researcher's responsibility to test the tools to establish that the data collected based upon the tools used can be trusted. This means the researcher must demonstrate that the measurement tools are both valid and reliable so the results can be believed.

LINKS TO LEARN MORE

Reliability & validity: https://www.youtube.com/watch?v=9ltvDNAsO-I

References

Converge. (n.d.). *Merriam-Webster.com*. Retrieved from https://www.merriam-webster.com/dictionary/research

Crocker, L. M., & Algina, J. (1986). *Introduction to classical and modern test theory*. New York, NY: Holt, Rinehart, & Winston.

Nimon, K., Zientek, L. R., & Henson, R. K. (2012). The assumption of a reliable instrument and other pitfalls to avoid when considering the reliability of data. *Frontiers in Psychology, 3*, 102. doi:10.3389/fpsyg.2012.00102

Trochim, W. M. K., Donnelly, J. P., & Arora, K. (2016). *The research methods: The essential knowledge base* (2nd ed.). Boston, MA: Cengage Learning.

Van Dam, N. T., & Earleywine, M. (2011). Validation of the Center for Epidemiologic Studies Depression Scale-Revised (CESD-R): Pragmatic depression assessment in the general population. *Psychiatry Research, 186*(1), 128–132. doi:10.1016/j.psychres.2010.08.018

Wallach, M., & Kogan, N. (1965). *Modes of thinking in young children. A study of the creativity-intelligence distinction*. New York, NY: Holt, Rinehart, & Winston.

Webb, N. M., Shavelson, R. J., & Haertel, E. H. (2006). 4 reliability coefficients and generalizability theory. *Handbook of Statistics, 26*, 81–124. doi:10.1016/S0169-7161(06)26004-8

Young, Q.-R., Nguyen, M., Roth, S., Broadberry, A., & Mackay, M. H. (2015). Single-item measures for depression and anxiety: Validation of the Screening Tool for Psychological Distress in an inpatient cardiology setting. *European Journal of Cardiovascular Nursing, 14*(6), 544–551. doi:10.1177/1474515114548649

10

From Population to Sample

INTRODUCTION, or *Finding the right subjects for a research study*

A group of subjects, derived from a larger population, will be identified in a quantitative research project as the sample. A qualitative researcher might identify specific characteristics desired in a subject and use just that one person (or a limited number of subjects) while diving deeply into the phenomenon of interest. The process that a researcher uses to move from identifying a population to selecting a sample, or specific subjects, follows principles and strategies. Each study must have a plan that will identify who (or, in some cases, what) will be selected and observed or surveyed as part of the quest to answer the research question. This chapter presents the most common kinds of sampling used in research studies.

You have been thinking about the Big Problem since the start and identified the discrepancy early on, so you probably already have an idea about who (or what) you need information from for your study. The whole idea behind identifying a sample is to be able to produce answers to the research question through testing a group that is representative of the group of interest. This chapter outlines the process of choosing the sample, taking into consideration the different categories of samples and explaining how to develop a sample plan that will be right for your study. In sampling it is not that one kind of sample is better than another, rather the goal is to identify the best sample that represents the population of interest to answer or shed light on the research question.

OBJECTIVES

In this chapter you will learn about:

- The principles of sampling
- The principles of probability and nonprobability
- Sample size
- Sampling in quantitative studies
- Sampling in qualitative studies

IMPORTANT DEFINITIONS

Some of the important vocabulary for this chapter include the following:

Population: All these people (or things) fit the description of who would be of interest to your study, based upon the aim/purpose and research question.

Target Population: All these people (or things) fit the description of who would be of interest to your study, based upon the aim/purpose and research question—and who would be available for your study.

Sample: This subgroup includes people, things, or events that will be examined by your study and is taken from the target population.

Element: The element in a sample is a single unit, which might be a person, a place, or a thing, depending on what the researcher is sampling.

Representativeness: This is a quality of the sample indicating that it resembles the target population, which is a representative of the population of interest. The representativeness of a sample indicates that the characteristics of the sample reflect the characteristics of the population and so the results (depending on a few other factors like power) might be generalizable to the larger population.

Probability Sample (*Quantitative Studies*): The subjects in a probability sample fit a sampling frame, which identifies *all* the criteria or elements desired in a sample. In this way everyone would have an equal chance to be selected for the study.

Nonprobability Sample (*Quantitative Studies*): The subjects in a nonprobability sample will have the criteria or elements that are available, rather than all that are desired. By specifying the available elements, some subjects are automatically eliminated, so there is not equal probability of everyone having the same chance to be selected.

Random Sample: These subjects are chosen for inclusion randomly; each subject has an equal possibility of being included. A random sample can be simple, systematic, or stratified.

Convenience Sample: This group of subjects is accessible to the researcher (convenient).

Purposive Sample: A group of subjects are identified because they meet a specific criterion that is important to the research study (e.g., pregnant women).

Snowball Sampling (*Qualitative Studies*): A subject is chosen because of characteristics of interest and is asked to invite others who are ready to volunteer.

Theoretical Sampling (*Qualitative Studies*): Qualitative research dives into the information from an individual participant or a small group of participants. It provides a depth of rich information that can yield greater insight or understanding of a phenomenon. The qualitative researcher will seek the element, or small group of elements, that can provide the richest information, rather than a large group whose responses could be generalized.

PRINCIPLES OF SAMPLING

Choosing a sample from which the researcher will obtain information related to the Big Problem and current problem at hand must arise from the aim of the study and reflect the variables in the research question. The choice of the sample (which can be people, places, events, or animals) can have an impact on the validity and reliability of the results of the study, just as the choice of a measurement tool could. It is impossible to get information from all elements (subjects) of a population—the full universe of elements—and so a sample representative (or some of the population) of that universe is mandated. The researcher must consider what characteristics are most important for the sample to have and, if conducting quantitative research, how many elements (or units) need to be included. If the researcher is engaged in qualitative research, the question of identifying the information-richest element needs to be assessed in order to collect the data that can provide the most evidence related to the phenomenon.

Fast Facts

Universe Population to Target Population to Randomized Sample

Marshall et al. (2011) wanted to uncover some information that could help reduce the level of freshman consumption of alcohol on college campuses through a social norms campaign. The population for that study purpose would be all freshmen students on all college campuses in the United States. Obtaining information from all of those subjects would be very expensive and time-consuming (and probably unlikely to ever happen).

Identifying one college campus that fulfilled the criterion provided a "target population." Then Marshall et al. (2011) identified freshmen living in school housing, for which there were two residence halls. A coin toss *randomly* determined which residence hall was the intervention hall (A) and which one was the nonintervention hall (B).

The Sample Plan

You have been invited to a "shoestring" potluck dinner. You might want to bring a large soup made of crab, lobster, and oysters. When you look around the grocery store, you find that there is no seafood available, nor is there any shellfish. To order these foods online would be extremely expensive. The dish you want to make is not really appropriate for a shoestring potluck dinner, the cost is high, and the nonavailability of the elements for the recipe makes the dish unfeasible. You needed a sampling frame that could help you list the items needed and a plan that would identify that the elements you chose for your dish were not ones that would be valid in the shoestring potluck.

Finding your sample needs to use the same commonsense logic that would be necessary for any endeavor requiring a plan in order to achieve success. Sampling is such an important aspect of a successful research study that it can sometimes make or break the study. It starts with defining what/who the important elements are and identifying the population (universe) that has those elements/subjects. From that population, the researcher identifies a target population, elements/

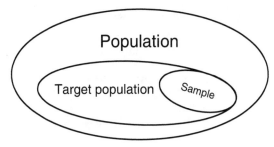

Figure 10.1 Finding the sample: From population to target population to final sample.

subjects that include the criteria of interest to study. From there the researcher moves to identifying accessibility: what/who can I have access to? See Figure 10.1.

Sample Frame: The sample frame should have all possible elements (subjects) that have the desired characteristics for the study that can be studied in the population.

N Versus *n*: In research samples the capital letter N represents the amount of elements identified in a sampling frame. The small italicized *n* represents the desired sample size.

Eligibility Criteria: Who should be included in this population/ target population and eventually sample? Establishing criteria makes it clearer to identify who/what should be considered appropriate for participating in this study. By setting up criteria for who can be included (inclusion criteria) as well as who should not be included (exclusion criteria), a boundary of sorts is established for choosing the elements. This process is true for research studies and also for literature reviews. The general topic looks at the universe of articles, and then the researcher identifies the target sample of accessible journals and applies the *inclusion criteria*: published in the last 5 years, only randomized controlled trials (RCTs), published in English, and focused on the topic (freshman alcohol consumption). *Exclusion criteria*: any school that is less than a 4-year college, any private college, graduate schools.

Minimizing Sampling Bias: Bias is when one group of elements, or a particular characteristic of a group, has more opportunity to be represented than another. A good example of a biased sample would be daytime, landline home calling polls because it limits the sample to only those people who are home during the day and who have landlines. People who have to work during the day and people who have given up landlines for cell phones would be excluded from this sample.

Keeping Ethics in Mind: Ethical consideration in conducting research and sample selection underscore the importance of examining the purpose of the research, demonstrating respect and justice for the participants and ensuring subject protection and transparency in both purpose and data collection. Ethical considerations related to all aspects of research is examined in Chapter 11, "Impact of the Outside World."

PRINCIPLES OF PROBABILITY AND NONPROBABILITY SAMPLING

Probability Sampling

When all the elements are included in a sample frame, and each one of those elements has an equal opportunity to be included in the final sample, a probability sample is obtained. It is the random selection of elements from a sample frame that is indicative of a probability sample. For those researchers who are seeking to recruit a probability sample, this Fast Facts book should be only one of many books they can use to guide them in their research. This brief explanation will not provide sufficient information for engaging in probability sampling techniques. Advantages: eliminates bias, more credible. Disadvantage: complicated implementations.

Ensuring Randomness *Selection in a Sample*

There are a couple of ways to assure that the final sample was chosen randomly (see Table 10.1). One way is to use a table of random numbers, which can be found online, in most statistic textbooks, and in some nursing research textbooks. Another method might use a computer program that generates a sample from the elements put in a file, or even just pulling names out of a hat can provide a random sample. Remember that random means that each element has an equal opportunity to be chosen as the next.

Nonprobability Sampling

This type of sampling, unlike the probability sampling, does not assure that each element in the sample frame has an equal chance of being selected and so might not be as representative as the probability sample. Nonprobability sampling also does not require establishing a sample frame (see Table 10.2). Advantage: easier to implement. Disadvantage: more likely to have bias.

Table 10.1

Probability Sampling: Methods and Techniques to Ensure Randomness

Probability Sampling	Explanation	Technique
Simple random	There is random selection of all the elements from a sample frame.	Number all elements in sample frame and randomly select elements using a random technique.
Systematic random	The elements are grouped together (listed) in no specific way, and a systematic choice is made to identify the sample.	The systematic random sample looks at the sample that is available and the number needed for the study, dividing the full number by the desired n to see how many times that n goes into the full sample (x). The list of the sample is made up, and then randomly start somewhere in the list. Example: You have 300 in the sample set, you want 25 in the sample, 300/25=12, so you take every 12th element for the sample.
Stratified random	By utilizing segments of a population that fit a criteria, different types of stratified samples can be generated. See Figure 10.2a.	The strata are defined first and divided into sampling frames. Then a simple or systematic sampling approach is applied.
Cluster sampling/ multistage sampling	When the desired sample is too geographically scattered, multiple (two or more) random sampling is done with groups (or clusters) in two or more stages. The random selections start from the largest group and continue until the unit of sampling. See Figure 10.2b.	After identifying the target population, randomly identify geographic areas, like states (e.g., choose three states)—further stratify to towns (randomly select five towns), randomly select 10 smaller units (e.g., schools), and finally randomly identify units (e.g., 15 students from each school).

Source: Adapted from Norwood, S. (2010). *Research essentials foundations for evidence based practice* (pp. 230–233). Boston, MA: Pearson.

Table 10.2

Nonprobability Sampling: Methods and Techniques

Nonprobability Sampling	Explanation	Technique
Convenience (available) sample	The researcher has access to this sample when collecting data (e.g., a professor's classroom or a healthcare worker's hospital).	Utilize the elements that are conveniently available at the time of research. To randomize, either apply simple random sampling technique to the N to achieve a randomized n, or choose to include every xth element from a group arriving for sampling.
Purpose/criterion (judgment) sampling	Utilize a specific sample of elements that are chosen specifically based on criteria or characteristics (e.g., females with opioid use disorder). This approach often is used to pretest study procedures or measurement instruments.	Identify specific criteria required for study investigation and include only those who reflect this identified criteria. *Often used in qualitative studies*
Network/snowball sampling	Elements who are recruited are asked to refer others sharing common characteristics to volunteer to participate. The initial elements are included by purposive sampling techniques or referral/ nomination.	After recruiting initial elements for the study, the participants refer others who have characteristics like themselves, for the study. *Often used in qualitative studies*
Quota sampling	A quota refers to a fixed number of characteristics (gender, age, etc.) that are needed in the elements identified to be included in the study.	List the characteristics of interest and divide them into groups. Identify how many from each group is needed/ desired and then identify a convenience sample from which to fill the group quotas.

(continued)

Table 10.2

Nonprobability Sampling: Methods and Techniques (*continued*)

Nonprobability Sampling	Explanation	Technique
Systematic	Using a convenience sample, take a portion of the elements.	Systematically take every xth element in a convenience sample.

Source: Adapted from Norwood, S. (2010). *Research essentials foundations for evidence based practice* (pp. 233–234). Boston, MA: Pearson and Wood, M. J., & Ross-Kerr, J. C. (2011). *Basic steps in planning nursing research* (7th ed., pp. 161–163). Sudbury, MA: Jones & Bartlett.

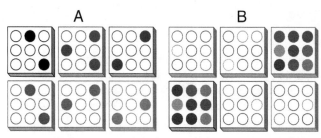

Figure 10.2 Difference between stratified and cluster samples. (A) Stratified sample. (B) Cluster sample.

Does Size Matter?

If a researcher is conducting a quantitative study, yes, the size of the sample matters a lot—the bigger, the better! If the researcher is conducting a qualitative study, the size matters, but just in so much as it can be a small size, even just a sample of 1. In this section sample size, as related to quantitative research, will be examined.

The first principle is the idea of randomness—the bigger the sample, the more likely the researcher will achieve the effect of randomness and deliver a result that provides an estimate of the population. The smaller the sample is, the more likely that the results will incorporate an error and not be a good reflection of the population of interest. The small sample increases the likelihood that the results do not relate to the larger group, so the conclusion cannot be generalized.

Determining how big a sample would be needed is always a conundrum for new researchers. Finding the right sample size for random sampling must be conducted by estimating the population size and also indicating how much error is acceptable to the researcher. The Central Limit Theorem (CLT) is a theory that provides a mathematical theory to test a hypothesis. According to CLT there is a rule of thumb that an *n* of approximately 30 randomly drawn from a population with a normal curve will be sufficient.

> In practice, some statisticians say that a sample size of 30 is large enough when the population distribution is roughly bell shaped. Others recommend a sample size of at least 40. But if the original population is distinctly not normal (e.g., is badly skewed, has multiple peaks, and/or has outliers), researchers like the sample size to be even larger.
>
> *Source:* StatTrek. (n.d.). *Sampling distributions*. Retrieved from https://stattrek.com/sampling/sampling-distribution.aspx

Links to videos and articles related to statistically determining sample size for a research project can be found at the end of this chapter. Table 10.3 provides a sample size estimator.

If you are wondering now about sample sizes, it is normal. It can be confusing, but here are some things to keep in mind as you consider the sample you will use for your study: Is your study qualitative or quantitative? Is the research being done as part of a class assignment, a thesis, or a DNP project? If it is being done as a requirement for a specific degree, check with your professor or adviser for guidance on what sample size is expected and acceptable. Are you repeating a study that has been done before? If you are, find out how many elements were used in that study, and use the original study as a guide. Is the study you are conducting a pilot study? A pilot study is a prestudy that examines the feasibility of conducting the full study and typically uses a smaller sample. Finally, is there a high degree of difficulty in finding elements for your study that have the characteristics of interest? It is always good to remember that the larger your sample the more generalizable and precise the results will be. A larger sample will also provide greater statistically significant differences when you engage in your analysis of data.

For those who are using a qualitative methodology, make sure the criteria you are looking to explore in the study are specific and clear so that subject identification is unambiguous. Be as clear with your exclusion criteria as you are with your inclusion criteria. Purposefully select the element(s) in your study based upon the criteria, and determine if you are looking for subjects with similar experiences (homogeneous sampling) or those with very different experiences (variation sampling). Any method of recruitment of subjects in a qualitative

Table 10.3

Sample Size Estimator: Suggested Sample Sizes

N	S	N	S	N	S
10	10	220	140	1200	291
15	14	230	144	1300	297
20	19	240	148	1400	302
25	24	250	152	1500	306
30	28	260	155	1600	310
35	32	270	159	1700	313
40	36	280	162	1800	317
45	40	290	165	1900	320
50	44	300	169	2000	322
55	48	320	175	2200	327
60	52	340	181	2400	331
65	56	360	186	2600	335
70	59	380	191	2800	338
75	63	400	196	3000	341
80	66	420	201	3500	346
85	70	440	205	4000	351
90	73	460	210	4500	354
95	76	480	214	5000	357
100	80	500	217	6000	361
110	86	550	226	7000	364
120	92	600	234	8000	367
130	97	650	242	9000	368
140	103	700	248	10000	370
150	108	750	254	15000	375
160	113	800	260	20000	377
170	118	850	265	30000	379
180	123	900	269	40000	380
190	127	950	274	50000	381
200	132	1000	278	75000	382
210	136	1100	285	1000000	384

N, population size; S, sample size.

Source: Krejcie, R. V., & Morgan, D. W. (1970). Determining sample size for research activities. *Educational and Psychological Measurement, 30*, 607–610. Retrieved from https://home.kku.ac.th/sompong/guest_speaker/KrejcieandMorgan_article.pdf

study should be clearly described with details of the interview process defined in the proposal. This is to protect the rights and safety of the participants. Qualitative researchers need enough elements or subjects in order to reach saturation of the theme.

DETERMINING WHAT KIND OF SAMPLE IS BEST FOR YOUR STUDY

Now you must once again go back to the hourglass of your study. It is time to determine how exactly you will measure the answer to the question (see Figure 10.3).

Protecting the Participants

Most studies require participants, people who volunteer to be part of the researcher's experiment. It is important that those who participate understand the nature of the research, the level of their involvement, the extent that the research might impact them, and the effect that their inclusion in the study might have on them or others around them. While the researcher is seeking to learn about a specific phenomenon, using either qualitative or quantitative methods, the outcomes of those results reflect the participation of human beings who need to be included in the purpose of the study and warned about any possible negative effects that might occur. In order to protect the rights of the participants, researcher are required to submit the

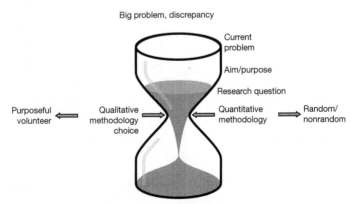

Figure 10.3 Hourglass of inquiry: Choosing how to measure the data.

proposal for a study to an institutional review board (IRB), which has as its sole purpose the protection of human rights for those involved in research studies. According to the National Institutes of Health (NIH), the IRB is "an administrative body established to protect the rights and welfare of human research subjects recruited to participate in research activities conducted under the auspices of the organization with which it is affiliated" (n.d.).

ROUNDUP

This chapter presented some of the sampling methods commonly used in quantitative and qualitative studies. The sampling method chosen by the researcher should be one that is practical, is appropriate to the research aim and question, and will provide reliable and valid data that the researcher can trust. Researchers must carefully plan the study's approach to gathering data, from identifying the measurement tools, establishing their validity and reliability, to having a sampling plan, obtaining IRB approval and then selecting and recruiting the elements. Lack of adequate planning in any of these areas can undermine the results of the study and render the endeavor unreportable. The well-planned proposal, however, sets a study up for success.

Fast Facts

Finding Your Sample

AIM/PURPOSE:_____

QUESTION:_____

My study will be using a qualitative/quantitative approach.

Qualitative: I am interested in looking at a *small group of people* and examining a specific experienced phenomenon with the aim of describing it in depth.

Inclusion criteria: _____

Exclusion criteria:_____

Method for identifying participants: _____

Quantitative: I am interested in identifying patterns, *using larger samples,* and predicting trends.

Inclusion criteria: _____

Exclusion criteria:_____

Method for identifying participants:_____

(continued)

(continued)

Quantitative	Qualitative
Identify element(s) from research question and aim.	Identify element(s) from research question and aim.
Establish inclusion and exclusion criteria.	Establish inclusion and exclusion criteria.
Identify method for recruiting a sample from the quantitative list.	Identify method for recruiting a sample from the quantitative list.
Discuss with supervisor/professor about the intended method for sampling.	Discuss with supervisor/professor about the intended method for sampling.
Apply for, and receive, permission from an institutional review board to continue to the next step of your study.	**Apply for, and receive, permission from an institutional review board to continue to the next step of your study.**

LINKS TO LEARN MORE

Types of Sampling Methods: https://www.youtube.com/watch?v=pTuj57uXWlk

How to determine the sample size for your study: https://unstick.me/determine-the-sample-size-study

Understanding the Central Limit Theorem: https://www.youtube.com/watch?v=_YOr_yYPytM

References

Krejcie, R. V., & Morgan, D. W. (1970). Determining sample size for research activities. *Educational and Psychological Measurement, 30*, 607–610. Retrieved from https://home.kku.ac.th/sompong/guest_speaker/Krejcieand Morgan_article.pdf

National Institutes of Health. (n.d.). *Institutional review board*. Retrieved from https://grants.nih.gov/grants/glossary.htm#InstitutionalReviewBoard (IRB)

Norwood, S. (2010). *Research essentials foundations for evidence based practice*. Boston, MA: Pearson.

StatTrek. (n.d.). *Sampling distributions*. Retrieved from https://stattrek.com/sampling/sampling-distribution.aspx

Wood, M. J., & Ross-Kerr, J. C. (2011). *Basic steps in planning nursing research* (7th ed.). Sudbury, MA: Jones & Bartlett.

11

Impact of the Outside World: Legal and Ethical Considerations in Research

INTRODUCTION, or *The impact of worldly events on the validity of the results*

This chapter identifies two very important aspects of research that force the researcher to think outside the study to the bigger world and take into consideration responsibilities the researcher has to protect the subjects and understand how the real world can impact the study and its ability to be generalized. The first has two parts: the legal and ethical considerations that must be in every researcher's mind from the moment that a study is being considered. This aspect of a research study is guided by laws and principles of human rights that must be adhered to. The second is anticipation of the impact on the validity of the results by forces not necessarily part of the study. Research studies, not unlike the house we spoke of building in Chapter 5, The Theoretical Framework, need to take into consideration more than the blueprint. In order to be able to have a sense of security in the house, you must also know the seasonal weather, the neighborhood, and other things that could impact the home. So it is with a study, things like losing participants (attrition) or overtesting (test effects) can alter the results of the study in ways that could nullify the validity of the study itself. A researcher must know these guiding principles and mousetraps and plan the study diligently.

OBJECTIVES

In this chapter you will learn about:

- The ethical and legal guidelines to conducting a research study
- The threats to the validity of the study's results from inside the study
- The threats to the validity of the study's results from outside the study

IMPORTANT DEFINITIONS

Some of the important vocabulary for this chapter includes the following:

Ethics: Webster's dictionary defines *ethics* as moral values and principles guiding the conduct of a group. Ethics is considered to be a universal fairness when considering a narrow area of behavior, rather than a selective preference of what is broadly deemed as right or wrong.

Nuremberg Code: These guidelines were established after World War II in response to war crimes by Hitler. They are meant to assure that specific ethical characteristics of research studies are present, including consent, protection from harm, and a balance of risks and benefits.

Vulnerable Populations: These people are identified as requiring protection because of their age, life situation, or other factors that would deny them the full right of either ability to understand or ability to provide informed consent.

Common Rule: The Code of Federal Regulations (CFR) established federal rules reflecting the need for informed consent, institutional review board (IRB) approval, and specific guidelines for vulnerable populations. The common rule went into effect in January 2018.

Deception: Deception refers to the use of misinformation when recruiting subjects, which could affect their willingness to participate.

Assent: Assent refers to the agreement to participate from a person unable to provide legal consent. An example would be a child giving assent to participate in a study after the parents provided legal consent.

Consent: Informed consent is willingness to participate in an activity after being informed of all the risks and benefits associated with that activity. Consent is provided only by those who are over the legal age of consent, which in the United States is 18.

Proxy: Proxy is the provision of authority to be the representative of another person, for reasons of either voting or providing consent for inclusion in a study.

Internal Validity: The believability of a study is based on how well that study was conducted. A high internal validity implies that the effect seen at the end (dependent variable) is a real product of the impact of the intervention (independent variable) and not something else.

External Validity: External validity is the believability of the outcome of a study and the ability to generalize the findings to a larger or different population or different places or at different times.

PRINCIPLES OF RESEARCH ETHICS

What Is Ethics? How Is It Different From Morality?

Ethics is often confused with morality because both terms deal with values of right and wrong when considering behaviors and events. Although it is true that both deal with right and wrong or good and bad, morality usually is more personal and theological (religious) in nature, whereas ethics is more focused on codes of conduct of a social system in specific areas (law, research, medicine, etc.). Ethics in research establishes a nonjudgmental code of conduct that can guide biomedical research. It establishes the requirements set by society for fair and just treatment within a specific set of circumstances. Ethics usually governs the practice of professionals, guiding behavior through rules and laws.

Fast Facts

Ethics and Morality: A Story of Law, Ethics, and Morality

Mr. P, an attorney for JF, a healthcare provider accused of inappropriate contact with a patient, has taken the case as JF's defense lawyer. JF tells the attorney that the contact was professional and the other healthcare providers do not like that JF gives such personal care. Mr. P. discovers that JF has been let go from five other hospitals and nursing homes over the past 7 years.

(continued)

(continued)

> During the trial, Mr. P hears the testimony from coworkers, the patient's family, and even the patient, but the evidence is all circumstantial. Mr. P. has his own private beliefs on whether or not JF had inappropriate contact with the patient but continues to provide excellent legal defense and gets JF acquitted of all charges.
>
> ■ Is it ethical for Mr. P to represent JF? Why, or why not?
> ■ If JF engaged in inappropriate contact with patients, is it immoral and/or unethical behavior?
> ■ What is the ethics behind a jury being able to acquit JF of the charge, even if the patient stated it occurred?
>
> ✓ Mr. P, as a lawyer, has an ethical obligation to defend his client based on the evidence and according to the law.
> ✓ If JF engaged in the alleged behavior, it would be considered unethical, as it would go against the rules of providing safe patient care, and immoral, as it would violate social, and possibly religious, norms and also indicate that JF was lying to everyone.
> ✓ The jury must make a decision based on the evidence and according to the law.

Standards for ethics arose after World War II with the atrocities that had been done to those under the Third Reich's detainment, predominantly Jews. The Nuremberg Code outlines 10 mandates for ethical consideration during research, starting with voluntary consent as the first principle (*Trials of War Crimes*, 1949 as cited in "The Nuremberg Code," 2002). Following the Nuremberg Code was the Declaration of Helsinki in 1964, which delineated the differences between therapeutic research (when patients have a chance to participate in a study that can benefit their health) and nontherapeutic research, which is purely for the generation of new scientific knowledge, not necessarily for the benefit of those participating in the study (World Medical Association, 2019). In 1979, the Belmont Report was written to further the protection of human subjects following the discovery of the Tuskegee Experiments. This report focused on the therapeutic and nontherapeutic aspects of biomedical and behavioral research.

Protecting the rights of human subjects was not just an issue in the 20th century. As the world becomes smaller and our ability to reach into the lives of others through the Internet grows, updated, and sometimes new, guidelines are needed. One example of this is the Health Insurance Portability and Accountability Act (HIPAA; Public

Law 104.191), also known as the *privacy law*, protecting health data. Early in the 21st century a Presidential Commission for the Study of Bioethical Issues was commissioned by President Obama to look into issues of neuroscience, genomics, and protection of human subjects, adding 14 changes to the practices that were in place in 2011 (Presidential Commission for the Study of Bioethical Issues, 2011). The most recent change to the Belmont Rule, protecting human subjects, went into effect in 2018 and is called the *Common Rule*, which specifically targets protection for vulnerable populations. A link to each of these reports can be found in the Links to Learn More section at the end of the chapter.

Following are five studies that violated the rights of the human subjects. Can you identify how each took advantage of vulnerable populations?

Fast Facts

Five Unethical Studies: Nazi, Tuskegee, Willowbrook, Jewish Chronic Disease Hospital Study, HIV Studies on Kids

In World War II Hitler's Germany conducted experiments on *Jews and other prisoners* being held by the Third Reich in concentration camps, including, but not limited to, evaluating the effect of freezing temperatures on humans, surgery without anesthesia, and exposure to high altitudes. The subjects did not provide consent, and there were no rights afforded to them. Many of the subjects died or suffered permanent physical and emotional harm (Holocaust Encyclopedia, n.d.).

In America, from the 1930s to 1970s, experiments were conducted by the U.S. Public Health Service on *Black men* in Tuskegee, Alabama. Men were infected with syphilis and observed for symptoms over their lifetime for the effects of untreated syphilis. Even after it was established that penicillin would treat the disease, these men (and their wives and children) were not offered the drug (Centers for Disease Control and Prevention, n.d.).

A home for *developmentally disabled children* was the site for experimentation from the 1950s to the 1970s, where children were deliberately infected with hepatitis. Children would not be admitted to the home unless the parents gave consent for the experimentation ("Willowbrook Hepatites Experiments," 2009).

(continued)

(continued)

Twenty-two patients at Sloan-Kettering Institute for Cancer Research in New York City were purposefully injected with live cancer cells without consent and without the institutional review board (IRB) knowledge of the study. Patients, the doctors treating them, and the hospital were unaware of the study. When this study was made public, it was stopped, and the patients received appropriate care (Macklin, 2013).

Seven states in the United States conducted government-funded research on foster kids, predominantly minority, over a period of 20 years, causing physical and emotional distress and sometimes leading to death. Children were not provided with advocates, and many of the children died as the level of drugs given to them were typical of or greater than those doses given to adults (Solomon, 2005).

Ethical Principles

Research that includes human subjects is guided by three ethical principles (Figure 11.1):

- *Respect for persons*: People are autonomous and able to make free choices, unless they belong to a vulnerable population with diminished autonomy (e.g., children, patients, prisoners), in which case their rights must be protected by laws and other regulations. Avoidance of coercion (threats of harm or use of rewards for participation), use of misinformation, and covert data collection are prohibited as they go against self-determined, autonomous participation.
- *Beneficence*: This principle involves doing no harm to the participant and promoting any good that comes from the study. Beneficence always keeps the welfare of the participant in focus.

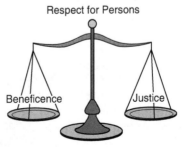

Figure 11.1 Balance of human research protection.

Harm to a participant can be in the form of physical, emotional, financial, social, or any combination of these four elements. Respect for the privacy of person and personal data fits under beneficence.

■ *Justice*: Justice involves the fair selection and treatment of subjects, including protection from risks. The inclusion and exclusion criteria of a study must be in keeping with the purpose of the study and supported by logic and evidence.

Informed Consent

Informed consent refers to the provision of characteristics of the study that a reasonable person would need to know in order to determine whether it is safe to participate. Projects and studies that include human subjects must also have a written consent form that provides the necessary information to the participant. Informed consent must include four features: disclosure (telling the participants what will be expected of them), comprehension (ensuring that the participants understand the information), competence (participants do not have diminished autonomy), and voluntary agreement (participation without coercion; Figure 11.2).

Institutional Review Boards

The IRB is an institutionally based committee where either the researcher works or where permission to conduct the study will be requested. The IRB committee examines the proposal to determine that the ethical principles are being applied and federal laws and guidelines for protection of human subjects are adhered to. The IRB can accept, amend, modify, or reject a proposal. The membership composition of an IRB board is directed by federal regulations. Those institutions that seek to obtain funding from the federal government are required to register with the Office of Human Research Protection (OHRP; U.S. Department of Health and Human Services [DHHS], n.d.) as well as acquire a federal-wide assurance (FWA; Grady, 2015)

The IRB has different levels of proposal review and determines which level is appropriate by following the common rule and other guidelines (Figure 11.3; DHHS, 2017). The levels are *exempt*: no risk assessed to participants; *expedited*: educational settings using educational tests, surveys interviews, or observations, benign interventions (e.g., game playing for knowledge gain); and *full board review*: any study with greater than minimal risk to participants. Each and every study *must* go through an IRB review, even if the researcher knows it will be exempt.

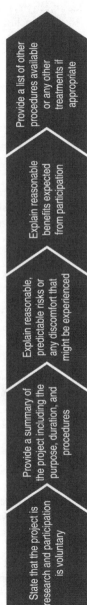

Figure 11.2 Informed consent procedure.

Source: Adapted from Chadwick, G. L. (2017). *Final rule material: Comprehensive guide to informed consent procedures.* New York: Biomedical Research Alliance of New York. Retrieved from https://about.citiprogram.org/wp-content/uploads/2018/07/Final-Rule-Material-Comprehensive-Guide-to-Informed-Consent-Changes.pdf

IRB Levels of Review

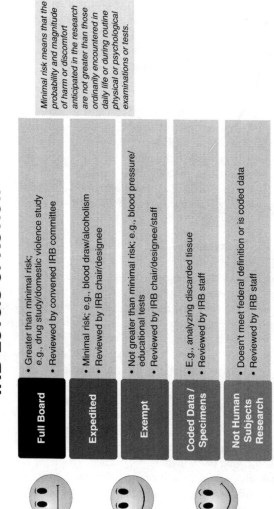

Full Board
- Greater than minimal risk; e.g., drug study/domestic violence study
- Reviewed by convened IRB committee

Expedited
- Minimal risk; e.g., blood draw/alcoholism
- Reviewed by IRB chair/designee

Exempt
- Not greater than minimal risk; e.g., blood pressure/educational tests
- Reviewed by IRB chair/designee/staff

Coded Data / Specimens
- E.g., analyzing discarded tissue
- Reviewed by IRB staff

Not Human Subjects Research
- Doesn't meet federal definition or is coded data
- Reviewed by IRB staff

Minimal risk means that the probability and magnitude of harm or discomfort anticipated in the research are not greater than those ordinarily encountered in daily life or during routine physical or psychological examinations or tests.

Figure 11.3 Levels of institutional review board (IRB) review.

Source: University of Southern California. (n.d.). *New Common Rule (IRB regulations): USC implementation.* Retrieved from https://oprs.usc.edu/policies-and-procedures/newrule

The protection of human subjects is of vital importance to every project and study that a researcher will conduct. Misconduct (intentional protocol breaches, falsification of data or results, plagiarism, and fabrication of information) on the part of the researcher can result in loss of funding, retraction of articles, and in cases of academic work, failure and expulsion from a program. The impact on care delivery from research misconduct can impact the kind of care that is considered evidence-based and could cause harm to the public.

Evaluating the published research you base your study on is also important in this arena. The inclusion of IRB approval in a publication usually means that the study followed ethical guidelines and the IRB found the researchers to be qualified to conduct the study. It is also to look at each article to see if there is a sponsorship for the study and if that sponsorship could be an influencing factor in the outcome of the study. Ethical issues should be a consideration for the researcher from the first thought of the Big Problem through the reporting of results and conclusion (Figure 11.4).

It is only after the IRB approval has been obtained that the researcher (you!) can begin the actual study and collection of data.

PRINCIPLES OF INTERNAL AND EXTERNAL VALIDITY

Following the guidelines to construct an ethical research study is very important. Determining that the subject you are studying is one that will not place your participants at risk and that their participation is autonomous with informed consent will allow you to achieve IRB approval and begin the collection of data. Neglecting to ascertain the protection of human subjects and the ethical soundness of a project is not the only pitfall that can undermine a study, however. The discussion of reliability and validity regarding data was the focus of Chapter 9, "Reliability and Validity." There are two more aspects of validity that need to be considered: threats to the internal and external validity of the study. These threats can be specific to the method (qualitative or quantitative) as well as the participant selection. A threat is something that will make the public question the conclusion of the study and reduce the ability of the researcher to generalize the findings to other samples. This section will introduce the threats that can impact a study's generalizability.

External Validity

When a person embarks on the research study journey, there is a belief that the results of the study will help to answer the research

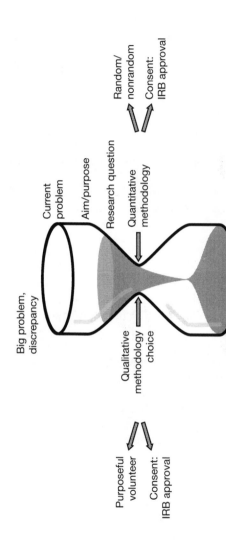

Figure 11.4 Hourglass of inquiry: Considering ethical issues.

IRB, institutional review board.

question and provide a possible solution to or explanation of the Big Problem. It is imperative, then, to make every effort to control any threat that could endanger the trustworthiness of the conclusion. A threat to the external validity (truthfulness) *in a quantitative study* can occur at the stage of choosing the design, establishing construct validity (see Chapter 9, "Reliability and Validity") to looking at how the intervention, setting, and history itself can affect the findings. Three main areas examine threats to design validity: (1) interaction of the selection of participants with the intervention, wherein those volunteering to participate are very different from those who do not, impacting the results of the study; (2) interaction between the intervention and the setting, wherein just the actual choice of setting has an impact on the willingness of participants to join the study; and (3) interaction of the intervention and data collection and events occurring in real-time history that impact the study results.

Another threat to the external validity of a study can be the impact of the researcher's expectations (*experimenter expectancy*), placing a bias into the data by having the researcher collect the information in a way that can impact responders. This is also called the Rosenthal Effect, after Dr. Robert Rosenthal, who conducted multiple studies demonstrating this effect. For example, in one of his famous studies (Rosenthal & Fode, 1963), half of the experimenters were told the rats were bred to be particularly intelligent, while half were told the rats were bred to be dull (in reality, the rats were all standard lab rats and not specially bred one way or the other). In learning trials, the "bright" rats outperformed the "dull" rats. Several methods can be instituted to avoid the Rosenthal Effect: have a different person than the researcher collect the data, use double-blinded groups so that the researcher or the participants do not know which group is getting the intervention, or minimize the interaction between the researcher and the participant by using written instructions, videos, online material, and the like. Table 11.1 describes the other external threats to validity in quantitative method studies.

External Validity Specific to Qualitative Research

When validity is discussed related to qualitative studies, the question of appropriateness must be considered in regard to the tools, the process, and the data collected (Leung, 2015). Samples are usually small in qualitative studies, so the procedures and methods to identify whether a systematic, purposeful, or adaptive (theoretical) method would be utilized. Methods that the researcher will use to extrapolate and analyze the data should also be clearly identified with documentation of all processes and materials collected.

Table 11.1

Threats to External Validity in Quantitative Method Studies

External Threat to Validity: *Antidote*	Definition
1. Sample or selection bias: *Randomization* 1a. Interactional effect: *Randomization*	1. No randomization of elements/subjects so that the final sample may not represent the population. 1a. Interactional effects of measurement tool or intervention, usually due to sample bias.
2. Reactive or interaction effects of testing/test effect/ pretest sensitization: *Eliminate pretest or use unobtrusive measures* 2a. Obtrusiveness of measurement: *Conduct study in a natural environment (field experiment)* *Use one-way mirrors*	2. When a pretest is given, it can affect the response of the participants, increasing their awareness to the construct of interest; for example, women were tested as to the importance of vegetables in a meal, prior to watching a video on cooking veggies. The women might pay more attention as a result of the pretest. 2a. When the impact on the consciousness and then the response of the participant are not due to a pretest but due to the exposure to a measurement tool or an experimental setting.
3. Reactive effects of arrangements: *Field experiment*	3. Participants in an experimental environment so different from reality know that they are being tested, impacting their responses.
4. Multiple treatment interference: *Single treatment design*	4. When more than one treatment is given during a study, it is hard to determine which treatment actually effected the results. This would limit the generalizability of the results.

Internal Validity

Internal validity reflects the believability that the effects being recorded actually reflect the impact of the independent variable (intervention) on the dependent variable (response). Internal validity is especially important when the researcher is trying to establish a cause and effect from the project. It is a reflection on the design of the study and the extent to which the researcher can control the independent variables. The first question to ask yourself is "Is there another reason or reasons that this outcome could have been achieved besides this intervention?" Often there are other reasons that the researcher might not have considered, being so focused on the research project's intention. Two types of variables that can cause this threat are confounding variables and extraneous variables.

- *Extraneous variable:* Any variable that might come into competition with the identified independent (acting) variable causing the actual dependent (outcome) variable
- *Confounding variable:* The variable, which is an extraneous variable, actually influencing the dependent variable and so the outcome of the study

Outcomes from threats to the internal validity of a study can result in the researcher believing there is an effect when there really is not one (false positive) or that there is no effect when actually there is (false negative).

Some of the factors that can impact the internal validity of a study are sample selection and group assignment, subjects leaving the study, events occurring in the environment of the study that could affect the responses of the participants, and the aging of the participants (they become wiser or change intellectually; see Table 11.2).

Internal Validity Specific to Qualitative Research

It is important to remember that there are philosophical differences between qualitative and quantitative research methods (Table 11.3). The validity in qualitative studies speaks to the researcher's ability to exert rigor and control in the study so that the results are accurate and truthful. If you recall, the objective in the qualitative study is to provide depth of understanding to a phenomenon through exploration of a participant's knowledge or experience. Establishing internal validity, therefore, would be focused on the participant rather than the researcher enforcing sampling controls and would reflect credibility, trustworthiness, and authenticity of results (Yilmaz, 2013). Credibility, rather than validity, would be demonstrated by the context-rich and detailed descriptions, the plausibility and comprehensiveness of the report, the existence of triangulation of methods to support the story, the consideration of rival explanations, and the acceptance of accuracy by the participants (or an explanation if there is not acceptance).

Rather than generalization, the qualitative researcher seeks to provide transferability, the ability to apply the results to other similar settings.

ROUNDUP

This chapter demonstrated the importance of remembering that the research study exists in the real world and needs to conform to

Table 11.2

Threat	Example
History	Events, other than the experimental treatments, influence results (e.g., a participant always arrives late to sessions or treatment).
Maturation	Participants experience changes (physiological or psychological) during the project (e.g., a participant experiences a death in the family during the study).
Testing	The effects of testing on the participant, which can cause testing fatigue or sensitization. Knowledge of being in a study (the Hawthorne effect) can also impact participant responses.
Instrumentation	When there is inconsistency in the measurement scales or the condition of testing. If there is a difference between the pretest and posttest, it might indicate a change in score that is not real.
Statistical regression	Statistically, when the subject's scores are very high or very low, there is a tendency to regress toward the mean during retesting, independent of the treatment effect.
Selection	If groups are not distributed randomly, there can be systematic differences between treatment groups.
Experimental mortality/attrition	Loss of subjects in a group or study that can impact results.
Diffusion of treatments	When participants of one group (control) are influenced by the participants of the other group (intervention).
Placebo effect	Knowledge of being in a study increases participant expectation, which in turn impacts results.
Contamination effect	Participants might start engaging in some activities.
Hawthorne effect	Participants enjoy the attention of the researchers, which can impact results.
Experimenter bias	An unconscious sway on the results due to the researcher's expectations and desires.
Interaction effects	A combination of any of the threats that impact the treatment variable.

Source: Adapted from Campbell, D. T., & Stanley, J. C. (1963). Experimental and quasi-experimental designs for research on teaching. In N. L. Gage (Ed.), *Handbook of research on teaching* (pp. 171–246). Chicago, IL: Rand-McNally, and Campbell, D. T., & Stanley, J. C. (1966). *Experimental and quasi-experimental designs for research*. Chicago, IL: Rand-McNally.

Table 11.3

Criteria for Judging Quantitative and Qualitative Studies

Aspect	Quantitative Terminology	Qualitative Terminology
Truth value	Internal validity	Credibility
Applicability	External validity Generalizability	Transferability
Consistency	Reliability	Dependability
Neutrality	Objectivity	Confirmability

Source: Adapted from Yilmaz, K. (2013). Comparison of quantitative and qualitative research traditions: Epistemological, theoretical, and methodological differences. *European Journal of Education, 48*(2), 311–325. doi:10.1111/ejed.12014, originally from Lincoln, Y. S., & Guba, E. G., (1985). *Naturalistic inquiry*. Newbury Park, CA: Sage.

standards, regulations, and guidelines of ethics as well as expectations related to validity of results. As a practitioner it is imperative that the "evidence" we are basing our interventions on can be trusted and that they have met the ethical guidelines, respecting the rights of the participants. When we look at the data quality, we are assessing the accuracy of the data, but when we look at the validity, we are assessing the integrity of the research. It is essential that the research we base our care on is free of bias and has passed the test of rigor and that the findings are credible. Whether we engaged in qualitative or quantitative methodology, the rights of our human subjects must be protected, and the researcher must be engaging in strategies, which can be incorporated into the study design, to eliminate threats to internal and external validity.

LINKS TO LEARN MORE

Videos

The Belmont Report's impact & importance: https://study.com/academy/lesson/the-belmont-reports-impact-importance.html

Institutional review boards (IRBs): https://www.youtube.com/watch?v=U8fme1boEbE

The Nuremberg Code. (1947): https://www.youtube.com/watch?v=WlV_aR4995I

Participating in research (Part 1 of 3): What is research? https://www.youtube.com/watch?v=4pLsHhP7yTw&list=PLrl7E8KABz1Ex7n0cjhxVgGDDF7xWHpF1

What's new in IRB review under the Revised Common Rule: https://www
.youtube.com/watch?v=zDsUUs9j3sQ
What is research ethics? https://www.youtube.com/watch?v=eweXtX8U7F8

Websites

Your rights under HIPAA: https://www.hhs.gov/hipaa/for-individuals/guid
ance-materials-for-consumers/index.html
Office of Human Research Protections: https://www.hhs.gov/ohrp

References

Campbell, D. T., & Stanley, J. C. (1963). Experimental and quasi-experimental designs for research on teaching. In N. L. Gage (Ed.), *Handbook of
research on teaching* (pp. 171–246). Chicago, IL: Rand-McNally.

Campbell, D. T., & Stanley, J. C. (1966). *Experimental and quasi-experimental
designs for research.* Chicago, IL: Rand-McNally.

Centers for Disease Control and Prevention. (n.d.). The Tuskegee timeline.
Retrieved from https://www.cdc.gov/tuskegee/timeline.htm

Chadwick, G. L. (2017). *Final rule material: Comprehensive guide to
informed consent procedures.* New York: Biomedical Research Alliance
of New York. Retrieved from https://about.citiprogram.org/wp-content/
uploads/2018/07/Final-Rule-Material-Comprehensive-Guide-to-Informed
-Consent-Changes.pdf

Grady, C. (2015). Institutional review boards: Purposes and challenges.
Chest, 148(5), 1148–1155. doi:10.1378/chest.15-0706

Holocaust Encyclopedia. (n.d.). *Nazi medical experiments.* Retrieved from
https://encyclopedia.ushmm.org/content/en/article/nazi-medical-experi
ments

Leung, L. (2015). Validity, reliability, and generalizability in qualitative
research. *Journal of Family Medicine and Primary Care, 4*(3), 324–327. doi:10
.4103/2249-4863.161306

Lincoln, Y. S., & Guba, E. G., (1985). *Naturalistic inquiry.* Newbury Park, CA:
Sage.

Macklin, R. (2013, February 5). Ethical controversy in human subjects
research [Blog post]. Retrieved from http://blogs.einstein.yu.edu/ethical
-controversy-in-human-subjects-research

The Nuremberg code. (2002). Retrieved from https://history.nih.gov/re
search/downloads/nuremberg.pdf

Presidential Commission for the Study of Bioethical Issues. (2011).
President's Bioethics Commission releases report on human subjects protection. Retrieved from https://bioethicsarchive.georgetown.edu/pcsbi/
node/559.html

Rosenthal, R., & Fode, K. (1963). The effect of experimenter bias on performance of the albino rat. *Behavioral Science, 8*, 183–189. doi:10.1002/bs
.3830080302

Solomon, J. (2005). Government tested AIDS drugs on foster kids. *NBC News.*
Retrieved from http://www.nbcnews.com/id/7736157/ns/health-aids/t/

government-tested-aids-drugs-foster%E2%80%8B-kids/#.XTcYMm
R7nct

Trials of War Criminals Before the Nuernberg Military Tribunals Under Control Council Law No. 10, October 1946-April 1949. (1949). Washington, DC: U.S. Government Printing Office. Retrieved from https://www.loc .gov/rr/frd/Military_Law/pdf/NT_war-criminals_Vol-II.pdf

University of Southern California. (n.d.). *New Common Rule (IRB regulations): USC implementation.* Retrieved from https://oprs.usc.edu/poli cies-and-procedures/newrule

U.S. Department of Health and Human Services. (n.d.). *Regulations, policy, & posting.* Retrieved from https://www.hhs.gov/ohrp/regulations-and -policy/index.html

U.S. Department of Health and Human Services. (2017). *Final revisions to the common rule: Protection of human subjects.* Code of Federal Regulations, Title 45, Part 46. Retrieved from https://www.govinfo.gov/content/pkg/ FR-2017-01-19/pdf/2017-01058.pdf

Willowbrook hepatitis experiments. (2009). Waltham, MA: Education Development Center. Retrieved from https://science.education.nih.gov/ supplements/webversions/bioethics/guide/pdf/Master_5-4.pdf

World Medical Association. (2019). *WMN declaration of Helsinki-Ethical principles for medical research involving human subjects.* Retrieved from https://www.wma.net/policies-post/wma-declaration-of-helsinki-ethical -principles-for-medical-research-involving-human-subjects/

Yilmaz, K. (2013). Comparison of quantitative and qualitative research traditions: Epistemological, theoretical, and methodological differences. *European Journal of Education, 48*(2), 311–325. doi:10.1111/ejed.12014

III

Test, Analyze, Discuss

12

Conducting the Research

INTRODUCTION, or *Steps to take before embarking on the research project*

You have now worked your way below the narrow section of the hourglass and chosen the method and design of your study. If you are engaging in quantitative research, you have gotten institutional review board (IRB) approval, chosen your setting, identified your reliable and valid measurement tool, recruited your sample, and developed a consent form for them to either sign or give passive consent, and now it is time to go out and start to gather the data. If, on the other hand, you are embarking on a qualitative research journey, you have identified your setting and the interviewee(s), as the interview is the most common mechanism for collecting the desired information. This chapter gives you an overview of conducting the research and collecting and coding the data. Note that the word datum *is singular and the word* data *is plural (American Psychological Association, 2010, p. 96). Plural nouns, such as* data, *are followed by a plural verb, so always state, "Data are" instead of "data is."*

OBJECTIVES

In this chapter you will learn about:

- Identifying the setting and the sample
- Data collection strategies: anonymous or confidential?

- Coding the data: quantitative and qualitative methods
- Storing the data: confidentiality

IMPORTANT DEFINITIONS

Some of the important vocabulary for this chapter includes the following:

Anonymous: Data collected from a participant can never be directly associated with that participant.

Confidential: Data are coded so that the identity of the participant is hidden, but the researcher can identify the respondent.

Raw Data: These data have been collected but have not yet been coded or analyzed.

Data Coding: Data coding involves assigning numbers, names, symbols, or abbreviations to represent themes (qualitative) or specific aspects of data (quantitative).

Coding of Survey Instrument to Protect Anonymity: By preparing the survey instrument with a code, rather than the participant's name, the information can be coded and the responses can be kept confidential. Anonymous surveys are also coded for analysis and review, making identification and review of outlier survey responses accessible by the code. Coding in qualitative research protects the interviewee, and coding of data in the interview allows for evaluation of interviewee's responses related to specific themes.

Bracketing: This process is used by qualitative researchers to reduce the possibility of tainting the results of a study with the infusion of personal bias (Tufford & Newman, 2010).

STARTING THE QUANTITATIVE AND QUALITATIVE DATA COLLECTION AND AVOIDING THE MOUSETRAPS!

Identifying the Setting and Sample

Face-to-Face Quantitative Data Collection

Consider back to your validity threats and do a check to make sure that the setting you have identified for data collection is one that will allow participants to feel free to accept or refuse participation without any sense of obligation. If you are a colleague or a professor and you are using a convenience sample that includes students or acquaintances, you might consider having the questionnaire/survey distributed by someone else. This will avoid the mousetrap of the participants wanting to please *you*, the researcher, and provide answers they believe you might want. Determine that the setting itself is conducive to distributing and collecting surveys/questionnaires, if that is the method you are using to collect data.

A questionnaire collecting data on behaviors might make people want to appear better than they are in reality—like responding with better parenting skills or healthier eating habits—rather than telling the truth. This mousetrap is called *social desirability*, meaning that participants try to make it appear to the researcher and others that they have the desirable characteristics that are being evaluated. The way to help avoid this mousetrap is to tell the participants before the survey is distributed that all the answers are combined and averaged with only group statistics (like percentages or averages) being reported, or to assure them that the responses are anonymous, not just confidential. Be clear that their specific survey will not identify anything about them personally.

Anonymity and confidentiality are very important in quantitative methods, protecting the respondent's right to privacy. The method of collecting data is the same; what is different is that the researcher does not know, and cannot find out, the individual respondent if the measure is done anonymously. This is especially important when collecting medical information, to ensure compliance with Health Insurance Portability and Accountability Act (HIPAA) regulations. It is important, when distributing the survey, to let the participants know that they have the right to turn in the questionnaire blank or to choose not to answer certain questions. This practice underscores the participants' right to autonomy.

A mousetrap for protecting anonymous data collection might be deductive disclosure, when the researcher can identify a respondent because of a specific characteristic like age, nationality, gender, or race. This can happen if there is only one person who is identifiably different in a demographic way, which would red flag the identity of that respondent. It is important to have a large-enough and diverse-enough sample to avoid this mousetrap. Ensuring a respondent's anonymity is part of beneficence (do no harm), an important ethical consideration for all researchers.

Collecting the surveys, if it is done in person, should also allow for confidentiality and anonymity. Placing a box or large envelope at the exit of the room where the surveys can be deposited is less threatening to the respondent than having to hand it in to a person, especially a researcher who is known to them. The envelope/box should be sealed if the surveys are collected by someone other than the researcher, to prevent the responses from being seen by those outside the study.

Digital Collection of Data in Quantitative Studies

Saleh and Bista (2017) identified online surveys as a current desirable method for data collection. Their study, which had a response rate of 78.9% ($n = 454$), identified that response rate for online surveys depended on the participants' interest in the subject, the way the survey was structured, how long the survey was, how the request(s) for completion was communicated to the respondents, and the assurance to the respondents of their privacy and the confidentiality of their responses. A mousetrap for online surveys can be the low response rate, for which Saleh and Bista (2017) identified two remedies. Male participants required reminders to participate, and participants who were older (no age specified) were more likely to respond when offered an incentive.

Advantages of online surveys include low cost, fast, and easy to administer and distribute. Disadvantages include antispamming software, fear of unsolicited emails, and refusal to open email from unknown senders for fear of malware, which reduces the response rate lower than face-to-face surveys. There are a couple of strategies that counter the mousetrap of low response (see Box 12.1). A researcher can target the sample to include those people with a higher interest in the topic or focus of the research (e.g., nurses for scope of practice for advanced practitioners). Keep it short and to the point to avoid attrition in the middle of the long survey! Usually under 15 minutes is the gold standard. Make sure that the opening invitation and the consent form (yes, online surveys require consent from the respondent) assure confidentiality of the information that will be provided to the researcher. When structuring the questions, keep them short and to the point, and be sure to use a professional voice when inviting participants (Saleh & Bista, 2017).

Data Collection in Qualitative Studies

The instrument for data collection in a qualitative study is usually the researcher. Problems can occur for the qualitative researcher when establishing a comfortable setting, during data collection, and even during data transcription. Setting is very important in the qualitative study so that the participant is relaxed, able to connect with the researcher, and comfortable sharing information. The setting should

BOX 12.1 ELEVEN WAYS TO INCREASE PARTICIPATION IN ONLINE SURVEYS

1. Use authority figures and organizations to distribute the survey (e.g., hospital).
2. Find a target sample that is interested in the topic of research.
3. Offer incentives.
4. Keep it short and simple.
5. Use a professional invitation that states how long it takes to complete.
6. Use closed-ended items; reduce the number of open-ended questions.
7. Make assurances of anonymity and confidentiality.
8. Explain the data collection, handling, storage, and disposal.
9. Make the invitations professional and personal.
10. Send a reminder (not more than three) for motivation to complete.
11. Respect the time constraints of the target sample, including time of year.

Source: Adapted from Saleh, A., & Bista, K. (2017). Examining factors impacting online survey response rates in educational research: Perceptions of graduate students. *Journal of Multidisciplinary Evaluation*, *13*(29), 63–74. Retrieved from http://journals.sfu.ca/jmde/index.php/jmde_1/article/view/487

be one that promotes the relationship between the interviewer and interviewee. The setting should also be quiet and free of loud noises and other possible distractions, allowing for a relaxed interview and a resulting clear recording or videotaping.

Qualitative research is laden with mousetraps due to its subjective nature. A researcher must engage in self-analysis to determine personal biases and beliefs that might impact data collection. It is important also to evaluate personal beliefs in the light of how they might impact the researcher's ability to impartially hear what the interviewee is saying in the interview as well as for the researcher to be aware of how those beliefs could color the analysis of the conversation. Awareness of the mousetraps, and engaging in strategies that can minimize them, can increase the study's trustworthiness.

The researcher should have prepared an interview protocol that describes the way the researcher will conduct the interview.

Instrumentation. During an interview, the participant may be recorded or videotaped, or the interviewer might take notes. Technological malfunctions during an interview can destroy the relationship built between the researcher and the subject, to say nothing of the wasted time and expense of coming to an interview. The simpler the technology, the less likely it is to fail. Capacity with easy-to-use technology that instantly records or tapes the interviewee verbatim must use a memory system that is both reliable and confidential. This is especially important today with the automatic uploading of voice recordings to "the cloud" from telephones and personal computers. Strategies to avoid malfunction of equipment include checking it in advance and making certain that it will not store information in the cloud.

Let the participant know how much time the interview will take so that plans can be made to be available for the whole session. If it is at the interviewee's home, request that there will be someone in the home who can field any interruptions during the interview.

Other mousetraps in transcription and analysis of data were identified by Easton, McComish, and Greenberg (2000) and are presented in Table 12.1.

DATA CODING

What Is Data Coding, and Why Is It Important?

Every researcher, whether using a quantitative, qualitative, or mixed methods approach, will have to code the data (information) collected in order to analyze them. A code simply means a symbol that represents something else. A taxonomy, or classification, is a method of categorizing verbal information in a specific topic, from which the researcher can develop or identify a conceptual framework. Without identifying taxonomies, misunderstandings can arise. At the start of this book, you were introduced to the taxonomy of research vocabulary, words that in other instances held different meanings but, when seen in the light of research, were specific and understandable. In qualitative research, the taxonomy must be specifically related to the topic of the research and the concept being analyzed.

A literature search into *research coding* reflects that coding is discussed more rigorously in reference to qualitative research. This might be because in qualitative research the raw data can be in transcript form from an interview or maybe a video or pictures, which need to be classified, organized, and analyzed. The coding of information related to the concept of interest then, whether using a processing program or interrater reliability methods, highlights areas of interest and indicates possible delineation of key themes.

Table 12.1

Mousetraps in Qualitative Data Collection

Type of Failure	Explanation	Reparation
Equipment failure	Recording or taping devices	Check and recheck all devices Check settings on devices Use battery-driven devices in case of loss of electricity Have extra batteries on hand
Equipment hazards	Conducting the interview where there is extraneous noise like pagers, loud speakers, or outside noise like construction or traffic	Prearrange that the interview setting is quiet Avoid the office (phone interruptions) and home (family/telephone) Place the recording device (or better yet use a microphone) near the participant
Transcription hazards	Inaccurate punctuation and mistyped words that alter the sentence's meaning; misunderstanding, mishearing, or misinterpreting a word or phrase Jargon and language differences or barriers	The researcher is the interviewer and the transcriber Always check the tape and compare to the transcription Employ professional transcribers (like court transcribers) Use italics and exclamation points to emphasize words and phrases

Source: Adapted from Easton, K. L., McComish, J. F., & Greenberg, R. (2000). Avoiding common pitfalls in qualitative data collection and transcription. *Qualitative Health Research, 10*(5), 703–707. doi:10.1177/104973200129118651

The original data in quantitative research might be results from questionnaires, and in qualitative research, they might be transcripts, which are considered raw data. This raw data require transformation into data that can be categorized, evaluated, and analyzed. Coding requires the researcher to have a systematic approach to data collection, assisting to break down the data into smaller parts while also providing labels for those parts. Without labeling what the raw data are representing, it is very hard to start to identify trends, patterns, or relationships. Each category will have a specific code, allowing the researcher to put all the information from the category under that code. Depending upon the kind of research being done, the kind of coding system will be different. For example, the person engaging in qualitative research will have a specific philosophical approach that is accompanied by methodological style of data review. For the quantitative researcher, it is imperative to determine the type of data that have been collected, whether they are normative or nonnormative, which will guide the researcher into the correct statistical data analysis.

In either case, however, the raw data will require organization and coding.

Quantitative Data Coding

The first stage of your data analysis in quantitative research is the preparation of the data itself, including cleaning the data and assigning codes to them (Norwood, 2010). Sit down with a clean copy of the survey and set up the system of coding. If demographics have been collected, go through and assign numbers to the nominal and ordinal data (see Figure 12.1). For example, gender: 1 = male, 2 = female, 3 = transgender, 4 = other/prefer not to answer.

If age has been collected as ordinal data, an example might look like this: 11–20 = 1, 21–30 = 2, 31–40 = 3, 41–50 = 4, older than 51 = 5. Go through the full survey and code each question and answer; keep this copy as your guide for entering data at a later date.

Each of the surveys, when it is entered into the statistical package being used, must also be coded with a number. This is done so that if you need to come back to a specific survey, you will be able to find it. This is especially important if the researcher thinks that some data were entered incorrectly or data are missing. If data are missing from the survey, it is a good idea to give a specific number, like 999, when you are entering the survey into the software package. This way, when you start to look at the data to clean them, these missing data points will stand out, and you will be able to find the survey (because you numbered each one) and see whether data are actually missing or whether data were entered into the statistical package incorrectly.

All the data are coded, from the descriptive statistics that reflect the sample to the data from the questionnaires. This will allow the researcher to look at the sample for frequency distributions, measures of central tendency, variability, relationships, and inferential statistics (see Chapter 13, "Data Analysis").

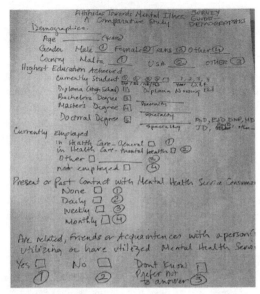

Figure 12.1 Coding a demographics sheet.

Note: **Age** (*ratio/scale*): In years. **Gender** (*nominal*): 1 = male, 2 = female,
3 = transgender, 4 = other/prefer not to answer. **Country** (*nominal*): 1 = Malta, 2 = USA,
3 = other. **Education** (*ordinal*): 1 = diploma/high school, 2 = diploma/nursing,
3 = bachelor's degree, 4 = master's degree, 5 = doctoral degree. (Specialty areas are
qualitative and are written in.)

Understanding the composition of the sample, its representativeness of the population, and the kinds of data that were collected
(nominal, ordinal, interval, or ratio) will help the researcher (and the
statistician if one is employed) determine the best route for analysis
of the data.

Qualitative Data Coding

The data collected in a qualitative research project include the
aspect of self-disclosure related to possible biases. Unlike quantitative research designs, there is not a clear-cut distinction between the
data collection and the analysis, because in qualitative research the
researcher is thinking about the data even as they are being collected.
The reflection that the researcher engages in while listening to, or
observing, the phenomenon/event/interviewee begins the analysis process. The researcher might keep notes on the observations
occurring in real time; these are called *field notes*. These kinds of

reflections begin the consideration of emerging themes even before the transcription process.

Transcription Process

Conversations are transcribed word for word, usually triple spaced, allowing the researcher to put in comments. It is very important that the actual words that were said are the ones that appear on the transcription, so many researchers read the transcriptions while also listening to the audiotapes to assure maximum transcription integrity.

To maintain confidentiality and/or anonymity, the researcher might redact (blacken out) or eliminate any conversations that reveal names or places of the interviewee. Emotional responses that can be heard in the voice can be added to the transcript to give more depth to the transcription. During this phase, the researcher can review original thoughts and consider new ones while reviewing the tape.

Once the transcription phase is done, the researcher dives into the data and lives there for a while, reading and rereading the words, listening to the emotions, and reexperiencing the event. This is important because now the data need to be tagged and grouped. Tagging of data in qualitative research "refers to the process of selecting from an amorphous body of material, bits and pieces that satisfy the researcher's curiosity, and help support the purpose of the study" (Babtiste, 2001, p. 10). Once tagged, the data are labeled, either from something directly connected to the transcription or from something applied by the researcher. The label's meaning is important only to the researcher so that there is an ability to get back to the data during the analysis phase.

Next the researcher groups the labeled, tagged data, using categories or characteristics to put similar data together and begin the identification of recurrent themes.

Marshall, Bliss, Evans, and Dukhan (2018) utilized self-reflections from students participating in a 6-second auditory hallucination simulation to uncover themes of efficacy in increasing knowledge of auditory hallucinations and empathy for those with symptoms of psychosis. Their study was a descriptive content analysis that employed a qualitative software package that allowed them to review 200 self-reflections. The team of researchers established interrater reliability to identify themes, and then utilizing Atlas.ti 7 software to review the reflections, they were able to quantify the qualitative statements. This process allowed them to identify 153 knowledge statements, 158 empathy statements, and 301 instances demonstrating insight.

Identifying themes for analysis in qualitative research can be done by one or more researchers with or without the use of software. It is during the cognitive work of tagging, grouping, and labeling that the analysis of the data begins in qualitative research.

Fostering Empathy: Looking for Themes

Dr. Marshall and Dr. Evans, psychiatric advanced practice registered nurses, employed a 6-second auditory hallucination simulation in their clinical rotation. The question of the efficacy of this method arose, prompting the research question "What effect does this experience have on the level of empathy of the student participants?" Students provided written self-reflections after the experience, which were collected and entered into a qualitative software program.

Ten reflections were randomly chosen from 212, and three researchers evaluated them for empathy and knowledge, and any other themes that might emerge, establishing an 87% theme identification reliability. Eighty-five narratives were randomly chosen from the 212 samples for evaluation. Five themes were identified, coded, and tagged across the 85 reflections: insight, knowledge, empathy, professional commitment to engage in therapeutic communication techniques, and value in the experience.

METHODS FOR STORAGE

The storage of the data is very important because it not only protects the study's findings but more importantly protects the confidentiality and anonymity of the participants. Many times researchers are collecting papers (surveys) or recordings (audio and video), which need to be appropriately secured in storage. When consent forms are signed, it is important to maintain those records with all study documentation and treat them as confidential files. If there are DVDs, mp3s, memory flash drives, or external drives, all these must only be in the care of those who have been authorized as part of the study to handle them, and they must be kept in a secure, locked area. Passwords that allow access to any digital records must be guarded and not shared, especially in this era of hacking; researchers must take the utmost responsibility for maintaining the confidentiality of the participants and their records. The researcher is responsible to keep the records for the files and also for those who have access to

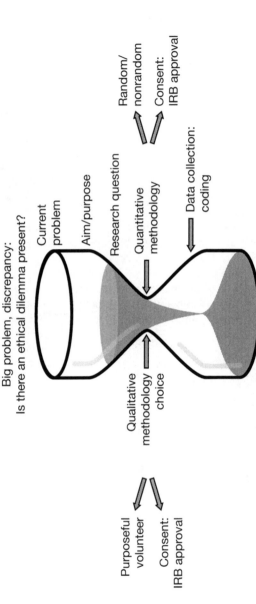

Figure 12.2 Hourglass of inquiry: Data collection and coding.

IRB, institutional review board.

the files. All persons working on a project must be trained according to the Human Research Training process demanded by the institution's IRB. Personal laptops and computers, especially those that automatically save to "the cloud," should not be used, and any person who has logged onto a personal computer for data entry must log out after doing the entry work, removing the flash drive on which the information is saved. Data that have been coded, copied, and saved for the duration of the study and according to the IRB must also be destroyed according to the IRB regulations. Raw data are usually kept on file for at least 3 years prior to destruction or according to the institution's policies.

ROUNDUP

Data collection, coding, storage, and destruction are all part of the research process. It is important that the process outlined in the IRB papers are followed and the data are securely stored and appropriately disposed of. This chapter provided a brief look at the possible mousetraps that a person might encounter when collecting and coding the data. It is the last stage prior to data analysis as seen in the hourglass in Figure 12.2.

In some quantitative projects, once the data have been collected and coded, statisticians might be consulted as to how to analyze the information. For both qualitative and quantitative study designs, data analysis, with interpretation of meaning and examination of patterns, is the next step.

LINKS TO LEARN MORE

Guidelines for responsible data management in scientific research: https://ori.hhs.gov/education/products/clinicaltools/data.pdf
Qualitative vs quantitative research: https://libguides.uta.edu/nursing research

References

American Psychological Association. (2010). *Publication manual of the American Psychological Association* (6th ed.). Washington, DC: Author.
Babtiste, I. (2001). Qualitative data analysis: Common phases, strategic differences. *Forum: Qualitative Social Research, 2*(3), Art. 22. Retrieved from http://www.qualitative-research.net/index.php/fqs/article/viewFile/917/2003

Easton, K. L., McComish, J. F., & Greenberg, R. (2000). Avoiding common pitfalls in qualitative data collection and transcription. *Qualitative Health Research, 10*(5), 703–707. doi:10.1177/104973200129118651

Marshall, B., Bliss, J., Evans, B., & Dukhan, O. (2018). Fostering transformation by hearing voices: Evaluating a 6-second, low-fidelity simulation. *Journal of the American Psychiatric Nurses Association, 24*(5), 426–432. doi:10.1177/1078390317750749

Norwood, S. (2010). *Research essentials, foundations for evidence-based practice.* Boston, MA: Pearson.

Richards, L., & Morse, J. M. (2007). *Readme first for a user's guide to qualitative methods.* Thousand Oaks, CA: Sage.

Saleh, A., & Bista, K. (2017). Examining factors impacting online survey response rates in educational research: Perceptions of graduate students. *Journal of Multidisciplinary Evaluation, 13*(29), 63–74. Retrieved from http://journals.sfu.ca/jmde/index.php/jmde_1/article/view/487

Tufford, L., & Newman, P. (2010). Bracketing in qualitative research. *Qualitative Social Work, 11*(1), 80–96. doi:10.1177/1473325010368316

13

Data Analysis

Katherine Roberts

INTRODUCTION, or *Figuring out what the data mean*

This chapter focuses on the different ways to analyze data, examining both descriptive and inferential data analysis. Researchers always work to make sense of their data through applying statistics, discovering what the data mean in the real world. Over the years, statistical analysis has become more sophisticated with the application of complex modeling; yet the basics have remained the same. These basics include the use of descriptive statistics. Some students learn how to use descriptive statistics in primary school, so it is likely that these types of statistics are somewhat familiar to everyone. The importance of descriptive statistics should never be underestimated! All research studies use descriptive statistics to describe the basic features of the data collected, even if it is a qualitative study. Descriptive statistics provide simple summaries about the sample and the data collected. In qualitative studies, the researcher still needs to describe the sample, and in many instances, qualitative data can be transformed into quantitative data (e.g., themes can be categorized and counted). Descriptive statistics differ from inferential, in that inferential statistics are applied when the data allow the researcher to draw some conclusions regarding the study's original hypotheses.

OBJECTIVES

In this chapter you will learn:

- The importance of descriptive statistics
- Which type of descriptive statistic to use with which type of data
- Types of inferential statistics
- The many different quantitative and qualitative statistical software packages

IMPORTANT DEFINITIONS

Some of the important vocabulary for this chapter includes the following:

Descriptive Statistics: The analysis of data (range, median, and mode) in meaningful ways

Inferential Statistics: The interpretation of data to draw conclusions about a population

Central Tendency: The center of the distribution of values

Mean: The average of scores

Median: The middle score of the range of scores

Mode: The most frequently occurring score

Range: The difference between the highest score and the lowest score

Variance: The spread of scores within a set of data

Standard Deviation: The spread of scores within a set of data by using the square root of the variance

Correlation: A measure of how two or more variables are related and the strength of that association

Regression: Assessment of whether changes in one variable predict changes in another variable

Statistical Significance: The likelihood that an effect is caused by something other than chance

Effect Size: The strength of associations between variables

Dispersion: How spread out the data are.

DESCRIPTIVE STATISTICS

When data are collected, the researcher receives raw scores (original scores that have not been transformed in any way). With raw scores, especially if there are a lot of scores, visualizing their meaning, or making sense of the data, can be difficult. Therefore, researchers will need to use *descriptive statistics* to interpret the data in a meaningful way. Through descriptive statistics, the audience is better able to understand what story the data are telling. Descriptive statistics are only used to describe; they do not allow researchers to make conclusions regarding hypotheses. Descriptive statistics include measures of central tendency and measures of dispersion.

Measures of Central Tendency

There are three ways of describing the central position of the distribution of values of the data; they are the mean, median, and mode.

The *mean*, or average, is the most common measure of central tendency. It is simply the sum of scores divided by the number of scores. For example, heart rate measures in beats per minute (BPM) were taken of nine patients, and they were recorded in Table 13.1.

To calculate the mean of this sample, you would add all the scores and divide by the total number of scores. In this case $82 + 74 + 63 + 61 + 74 + 52 + 48 + 70 + 42 = 576/9 = 64$. Simply stated, the mean BPM of the patients is 64.

The *median* is simply the middle score or the range of scores. To calculate the median, scores can be put in an order from low to high, and then the middle or center of the data range can be located easily.

Table 13.1

Sample Recording of Heart Rate in Beats per Minute			
Patient	Heart Rate in BPM (beats per minute)	Patient	Heart Rate in BPM (beats per minute)
Patient 1	82	Patient 6	52
Patient 2	74	Patient 7	48
Patient 3	63	Patient 8	70
Patient 4	61	Patient 9	42
Patient 5	74		

To calculate the median heart rate scores of the nine patients, the scores are rearranged in ascending order:

42, 48, 52, 61, 63, 70, 74, 74, 82

And then it is quite easy to see that the middle number is 63. The formula to calculate the median is to add the total number (n) of scores with 1 and divide by 2. With the nine patients the formula is $(n + 1) / 2 = (9 + 1) / 2 = 10 / 2 = 5$. So, the fifth value from either right or left of the ordered values is the middle number of 63. If there were eight patients instead of nine, the median is the average of the middle two values: 42, 28, 52, 61, 63, 70, 74, 78, so the median is $(61 + 63) / 2 = 62$. It is important to note that the median is unaffected by extreme scores or outliers. For example, in the case of the nine patients, if you had one patient who just sprinted up five flights of stairs and gets to the room with a heart rate of 137 instead of 74, the median is still 63; however, the mean would now be 71.

The *mode* is the score that occurs the most frequently. To calculate the mode, arrange the scores once again in ascending order—42, 48, 52, 61, 63, 70, 74, 74, 82—and then count how many times each score occurs. So, in this case all the scores occur once except 74, which occurs twice, and therefore, it is the mode. In some data, there can be two modes, which is called bimodal, or even more than two modes, called multimodal.

Acceptable types of data to compute the measure of central tendency are listed in Table 13.2 (see Chapter 8, "Methods of Data Collection," to review the different types of data collect to form quantitative measures).

Mode can be calculated for all types of data. Actually, it is the only measure of central tendency that can be used with nominal data. The median can be calculated for all except nominal data, which have no numerical order. The mean can be calculated only for interval and ratio data because only these types of data have equal distances between the values.

Table 13.2

Mode/Median/Mean and Data Types				
	Nominal	Ordinal	Interval	Ratio
Mode	Yes	Yes	Yes	Yes
Median	No	Yes	Yes	Yes
Mean	No	No	Yes	Yes

Fast Facts

Impact of Maternal Vaccination Timing and Influenza Virus Circulation on Birth Outcomes in Rural Nepal

Pregnant women between the ages of 15 and 40 were enrolled in the study with half receiving the flu vaccine and half receiving a placebo during pregnancy. Data were collected on birth weight, length of pregnancy, low birth weight (<2,500 g), if the birth was preterm, and if the baby was small for gestational weight at birth.

Results of Birth Weight Distribution

Birth Weight Measure	Placebo (n = 1,361)	Vaccine (n = 1,380)
Mean, g	2,762	2,804
Median, g	2,770	2,810
Range, g	820–4,420	1,260–4,800
Low birth weight	365 (26.8%)	315 (22.8%)

Simply by looking at the measures of central tendency (mean, median, interquartile range) related to the newborns' weights between the vaccinated women and those receiving the placebo, the effect on the fetus is clear. On average, those who received the placebo have lower birth weight babies compared to those who received the vaccine. However, we cannot determine if the results are statistically different from each other with just descriptive statistics; this is where inferential statistics comes in.

Source: Kozulki, N., Katz, J., Englund, J., Steinhoff, M., Khatry, S., Laxman, S., ... Teilsch, J. (2018). Impact of maternal vaccination timing and influenza virus circulation on birth outcomes in rural Nepal. *International Journal of Gynecology & Obstetrics, 140,* 65–72. doi:10.1002/ijgo.12341

Measures of Dispersion

Part of descriptive statistics also includes describing how spread out or dispersed the scores are. A number of descriptive statistics are available to describe the dispersion, including the range, variance, and standard deviation.

The range is determined by simply taking the highest score and subtracting the lowest score from it. In our example of the BPM of the nine patients, the mean score was 64; however, we know that not all the scores were 64: One was as high as 82, and one was as low as 42. The range would therefore be 82 − 42 = 40. One issue with range is that, similar to the mean, it can be affected by outliers, with outliers greatly exaggerating the range. Therefore, calculating the variance and standard deviation is useful because they can provide a more accurate and detailed estimate of the dispersion, or how much the data vary.

The variance and standard deviation measure how far the scores are spread out from the mean. Most researchers are working with a sample, not the entire population, so instead of calculating the population variance and population standard deviation, they calculate the sample variance and sample standard deviation. Researchers can calculate the variance and standard deviation by hand, which is easy enough to do, but most just use a calculator, Excel, or statistical program to calculate them.

To calculate the sample variance by hand, a researcher subtracts the mean from each score in the data set, then squares the sum of these, and divides by the total number (n) minus 1. For example, once again using the sample of the BPM of nine patients, starting with the first value of 42, the mean is 64, so the value 42 is 22 from the mean; square the 22 (22^2) to get 484. Continue doing this for each value and sum up all the squared results, which will give you 1,234. Then averaging this number would be 1,234 / (9 − 1) = 1,234 / 8 values, and you get 154.3, which is the variance. The standard deviation is just the square root of the variance. In this case it would be 12.4. A small standard deviation indicates that the values are close to the mean (narrow dispersion), while a large standard deviation indicates that the values are far from the mean (wide dispersion).

So now you should be able to understand all the statistics provided in the output in Table 13.3.

Table 13.3

Sample Descriptive Statistics of BPM	
Parameter	**Value**
Mean	64.0
Median	63.0
Mode	74.0
Variance	154.3
Standard deviation	12.4
Minimum	42.0
Maximum	82.0
Range	40.0

BPM, beats per minute.

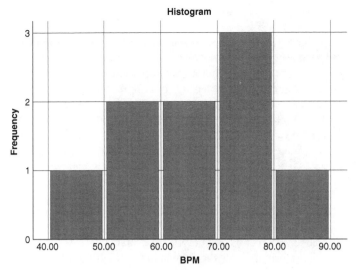

Figure 13.1 Sample histogram of BPM.
BPM, beats per minute.

Using charts and graphs can also help to provide a visual picture of the data (Figure 13.1).

When researchers use descriptive statistics, it can be helpful to summarize the data using either tables, charts, or graphs or written descriptions. If data are summarized in more than one way (written description and charts), it can be redundant for the reader. This is why journal articles usually display demographics in a table instead of describing the data in words.

There are many data visualization tools available to researchers that make the data look beautiful and stand out. However, many times beautiful-looking data are still hard to understand, and the story they tell is not clear. Researchers must choose how best to present their data that leads to clear understanding.

Fast Facts

Presenting Statistics Clearly

If you ever watch or read the news or even follow the news on social media, you will notice that broadcasters and journalists are consistently spouting out the latest statistics. Indeed, it is estimated that of almost a quarter of all news items contain at least one statistical

(continued)

(*continued*)

reference (Cushion, Lewis, & Callaghan, 2016)! However, sometimes the statistics that are presented within the context of the story are vague or imprecise. With the ever-increasing need to get the story out quickly, journalists may not have time to dive into the data, especially when complex statistical methods are used in the analysis. They may not even have the skills to be able to interpret statistical data and graphs.

The need to educate journalists to become more statistically literate is increasingly apparent; however, there are barriers to this, including the perception that it would be difficult to teach the material (Griffin & Dunwoody, 2016). This suggests that it is even more important these days for researchers to present their data in clear, meaningful ways with simplified language. Wider audiences, including journalists, will be able to accurately represent the findings and communicate them out to the public in a timely manner.

INFERENTIAL STATISTICS

Inferential statistics are different from descriptive statistics in that researchers use them to reach conclusions or interpret the data about a population based on the sample. Inferential statistics help researchers decide whether the differences between groups are strong enough to provide support for their hypothesis that group differences exist in the entire population.

Many different types of statistical tests are used to test hypotheses. Which test to use depends on types of data collected as well as the number of independent and dependent variables there are. Be aware that data can be analyzed in multiple ways, each of which could yield appropriate results. This book does not go deeply into the statistical analysis required for a thesis or doctoral-level study. Taking a statistics course can help you to determine which statistical tests to use. Also, there are a variety of online tools that can help researchers determine which test is the most appropriate (see Laerd Statistics in the Links to Learn More section). Those requiring more than descriptive analysis can also seek the guidance of either a statistician or a textbook that provides a deeper understanding of the analysis process.

Correlations

Correlations are used to determine whether an association between two or more variables exists and the strength of that association. A correlation coefficient is a statistic that describes how strongly variables are associated with each other. Pearson product moment correlation coefficient is used when the data are either interval or ratio. This coefficient is symbolized by the letter r and can range from 1.00 (indicating a perfect, positive, linear association) to –1.00 (indicating a perfect, negative, linear association). When $r = 0.00$, an association does not exist between the two variables. The closer the coefficient is to +1.00, the stronger the positive association is; the closer the coefficient is to –1.00, the stronger the negative, or inverse, relationship.

Predictions

Regressions are used to assess if changes in one variable predicts changes in another variable. Although regressions are thought of as predictor models, they do not necessarily involve predicting the future. Instead researchers fit a linear model to their data and use it to predict values of the dependent variable from one or more independent variables. When there is only one independent variable, the statistical model used is called a simple regression. When there are several independent variables, the model is called a multiple regression. Both correlations and regressions focus on the associations or relationships between variables.

Group Differences

Many study designs are set up so that researchers can examine differences between groups, usually groups of people. With these types of statistical tests, most often researchers are comparing the mean scores between different groups to determine differences. A wide variety of statistical tests can be used to determine whether there are differences between groups, ranging from between-subjects designs that involve independent groups to within-subjects designs that involve dependent groups, as well as mixed designs that have both independent and dependent groups. Simpler statistical tests involve testing for differences between just two groups. More complex designs can involve multiple groups, multiple treatments, and multiple dependent variables.

Fast Facts

Looking at the First Set of Statistics for Impact of Flu Vaccination on Fetal Development

The chart in Figure 13.2 shows the bimonthly mean birth weight in the placebo and vaccinated groups versus weekly influenza virus

(continued)

(*continued*)

circulation. Do you think any predictions might have been made from these data?

Significance Testing

Finding that an effect is statistically significant signifies that the effect is most likely not due to chance. The significance level is the probability of rejecting the null hypothesis in error. Researchers traditionally use either .05 or .01 significance level in their decision to reject the null hypothesis. A significance test provides a *p* value, representing the probability that random chance could explain the result. For example, a significance level of *p* = .05 indicates a 5% risk of concluding that a difference exists when there is no actual

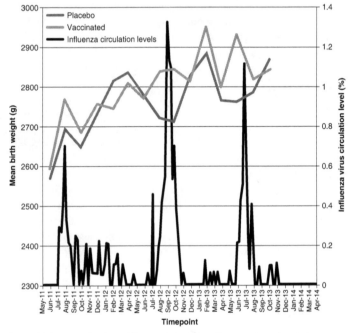

Figure 13.2 Mean birth weight in relation to influenza virus circulation.

Source: Kozulki, N., Katz, J., Englund, J., Steinhoff, M., Khatry, S., Laxman, S., ... Teilsch, J. (2018). Impact of maternal vaccination timing and influenza virus circulation on birth outcomes in rural Nepal. *International Journal of Gynecology & Obstetrics, 140,* 65–72. doi:10.1002/ijgo.12341

difference. Statistical significance does not tell us the importance of the effect or how large the effect is.

Effect Size

An effect size refers to the strength of associations between variables. An effect size is a standardized measure that is comparable across studies and not reliant on the sample size. There are several effect size measures, including Pearson's r and Cohen's d. To calculate an effect size, you can use one of the many online effect size calculators (www.uccs.edu/lbecker). A researcher will need to add in the means and standard deviations, and the calculator will compute the effect size. Some of the other effect sizes include Cohen's d, Glass's delta, Hedges's g, and odds ratio/risk rates. Note that effect sizes are not related to statistical significance. Statistical significance is about how confident the researcher is that an effect is real; it says nothing about the *size* of the effect. By contrast, Cohen's d and other measures of effect size are ways to measure how large an effect is.

Statistical Software Packages

There are many different statistical software packages that researchers can use that will provide both descriptive and inferential statistics. Microsoft Excel can perform some basic data analysis, such as descriptive analysis, but for more in-depth statistical analysis, it is recommended to use a statistical package such as SPSS, SAS, Stata, JMP, or R. Many health scientists use SPSS as their main package; however, R is becoming increasingly popular because this package is available free online.

SPSS: www.ibm.com/analytics/spss-statistics-software

SAS: www.sas.com

Stata: www.stata.com

JMP: www.jmp.com

R: r-project.org

For qualitative data analysis software, there are many software programs to choose from to code and analyze transcripts, field notes, videos, articles, websites, and so on; manage databases; and create data visualizations.

NVivo: www.qsrinternational.com/nvivo

ATLAS.ti: atlasti.com

Dedoose: www.dedoose.com

QDA Miner: provalisresearch.com/products/qualitative-data
-analysis-software

MaxQDA: www.maxqda.com

Most universities and colleges offer site licenses and provide researchers with instruction and even courses on how to use quantitative
and qualitative software packages. Therefore, before deciding which
package to use, investigate which ones are available and the cost and
time commitment needed to learn each program. There are also student prices for most statistical software packages as well as qualitative software packages.

ROUNDUP

This chapter provided information on the different ways researchers analyze their data to make sense of them. It demonstrated that
statistics in studies can be used to describe the sample, determine
relationships between variables, and, in some cases, predict outcomes. Kozulki et al. (2018) also demonstrate the need for honesty in
reporting statistics. Although their outcomes reflected a significant
increase in the birth weights of neonates whose mothers in Nepal
were vaccinated, the discussion stated the limitations that must be
considered when looking at the data, limitations that included the
use of a district with specific flu seasons, time of vaccination, and flu
exposure, and that they only looked specifically at birth weights and
term deliveries. Responsible researchers look at all possible reasons
for the results of the study, not just the one that was being examined.
They also do not exaggerate the results of the study and are able to
defend their research when it goes public.

LINKS TO LEARN MORE

Descriptive and inferential statistics: https://statistics.laerd.com/statistical
-guides/descriptive-inferential-statistics.php
*Laerd Statistics helps researchers learn more about statistics and the appropri-
ate statistical test to use:* https://statistics.laerd.com

Videos

Statistics intro: Mean, median, & mode: https://www.khanacademy.org/math/ap
-statistics/summarizing-quantitative-data-ap/measuring-center-quantitative/
v/statistics-intro-mean-median-and-mode

Type 1 errors: https://www.khanacademy.org/math/statistics-probability/
significance-tests-one-sample/error-probabilities-and-power/v/type-1
-errors

References

Cushion, S., Lewis, J., & Callaghan, R. (2016). Data journalism, impartiality
and statistical claims. *Journalism Practice, 11*(10), 1198–1215. doi:10.1080/
17512786.2016.1256789

Griffin, R. J., & Dunwoody, S. (2016). Chair support, faculty entre-
preneurship, and the teaching of statistical reasoning to journalism undergraduates in the United States. *Journalism, 17*(1), 97–118.
doi:10.1177/1464884915593247

Kozulki, N., Katz, J., Englund, J., Steinhoff, M., Khatry, S., Laxman, S., …
Teilsch, J. (2018). Impact of maternal vaccination timing and influenza
virus circulation on birth outcomes in rural Nepal. *International Journal
of Gynecology & Obstetrics, 140,* 65–72. doi:10.1002/ijgo.12341

14

Results: What Did the Project Discover? Why Is It Important?

INTRODUCTION, or *Where has this project taken me?*

Whether you have engaged in quantitative or qualitative methods to explore the discrepancy, identify the problem, and identify some evidence through the data, now it's time for the results. The results are the findings of your study based on the information that has been collected. For example, the actual words spoken in qualitative studies are the data that were collected related to a specific phenomenon, and the statistics that are reported in quantitative studies are related to that study's aim. These data are often presented in charts and figures, sometimes with an accompanying narrative. Looking at the results of a project/study is the most exciting moment! It answers the question "What did all that investigation turn up?" This is where the researcher determines how to make sense of what was discovered. The process of putting the results into a formula to report them helps the researcher identify any patterns or themes that have come up in the data. This chapter looks at how to examine the results and put them together in your report/paper so that you will be able to consider their meaning and whether what you have discovered is something that can change the way things are and move the world closer to how things should be (remember the discrepancy?).

OBJECTIVES

In this chapter you will learn about:

- Examining the results from qualitative research
- Examining the results from quantitative research
- Examining the results from a mixed method angle
- Writing up the results

IMPORTANT DEFINITIONS

Some of the important vocabulary for this chapter includes the following:

Normal Distribution: When a sample size is large enough, the distribution of the participants falls into a specific curve, which has a mean of 0 and a variance of 1 (see Figure 14.1). It is sometimes called a bell curve. Refer back to Chapter 13, "Data Analysis," for standard deviation explanation or Links to Learn More in this chapter.

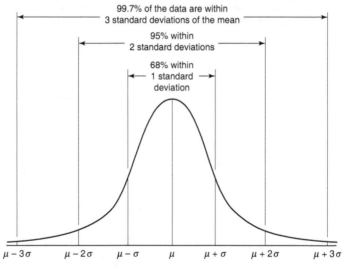

Figure 14.1 Normal distribution explained simply.

Note: μ, arithmetic mean; σ, standard deviation.
Source: Kernler, D. (2014). *A visual representation of the Empirical (68-95-99.7) Rule based on the normal distribution* [Image file]. Retrieved from https://commons .wikimedia.org/wiki/File:Empirical_Rule.PNG

Clinical Significance: Where statistical significance is looking at the probability of chance, the clinical significance looks at whether it is meaningful in clinical settings and practice. Sometimes statistical significance does not translate into a difference that can be seen in the clinical arena (e.g., pain relief).

Formulary: The formulary follows a format that crosses over from one study to another. The way to report the results in quantitative research often follows a formulary of providing the narrative of the demographics first, followed by an explanatory chart.

WHERE THE RESULTS FIT INTO THE RESEARCH PROCESS

Here it is again, the familiar hourglass of a research project (Figure 14.2).

REVISITING THE CONTINUING CASE OF JACK AND JILL

The truth is that the Jack and Jill research project/story is just that—a story, but let's consider for a minute that we all worked on the Jack and Jill study. In this chapter we will take it from the discrepancy to the results section (using facts that are just part of the story and not grounded in truth), looking at it from both the quantitative and qualitative approach (see Figure 14.3).

Only the Big Problem and the current problem are the same for both approaches.

BIG Problem/Discrepancy (*same for both approaches*):
Traumatic brain injuries (TBIs) can cause death and lifelong physical and emotional scarring. Children should be safe when

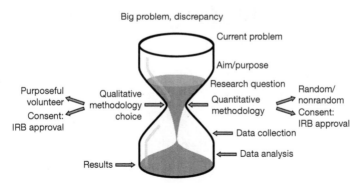

Figure 14.2 Hourglass of inquiry: Data analysis and results.

IRB, institutional review board.

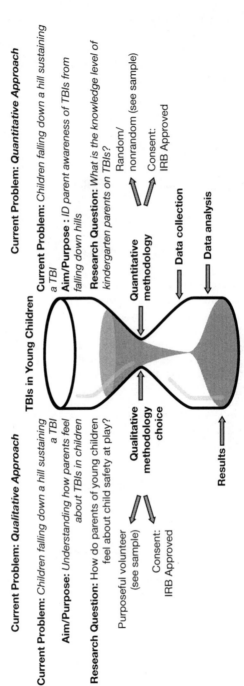

Figure 14.3 Hourglass of inquiry for the continuing case of Jack and Jill.

ID, identify; IRB, institutional review board; TBI, traumatic brain injury.

they are playing, but many children are not safe playing on steep hills and end up with TBIs.

Current Problem (*same for both approaches*): A neighborhood hill, which has a little well at that top where children play a game of fetch a pail of water, is resulting in increased TBIs in children under the age of 6.

The rest of the research project differs for qualitative and quantitative approaches (see Table 14.1).

Table 14.1

	Comparing Qualitative and Quantitative Approaches for the Continuing Case of Jack and Jill	
	Qualitative Approach	**Quantitative Approach**
Aim/Purpose	Understand how parents with children who have had a TBI playing on the hill with the well feel	Examine the level of parental knowledge of cause and impact of TBIs in young children
Research Question	How do parents of children who have sustained TBIs playing on the hill feel about TBIs in young children?	What is the level of parental knowledge related to the causes of and long- and short-term effects of TBIs?
Hypothesis	None	Parents with greater knowledge are less likely to have their children experience TBIs
Design	Qualitative, interview	Quantitative, survey
Setting	Pediatrician's office	PTA meeting in four elementary schools near the hill
IRB Approval	Approved prior to any data collection	Approved prior to any data collection
Sample	Purposive sample: Parents with children who have had a TBI Letter sent home to all parents of students at four elementary schools, explaining the project and requesting volunteers One parent from pre-k, kindergarten, first, second, and third grade chosen based upon availability; consent form provided	Purposive, nonrandomized All parents with children in third grade and under at four elementary schools will be provided with a survey when arriving for the PTA meeting, with a consent form and explanation of the study attached

(continued)

Table 14.1

Comparing Qualitative and Quantitative Approaches for the Continuing Case of Jack and Jill (continued)

Method of Data Collection	Videotaped or audiotaped interviews with five parents; notes taken during interview as well	Surveys distributed to all parents arriving at the meetings PTA president explains the anonymous survey and reason for study and tells parents that the surveys can be deposited in boxes located at the exit of the auditorium
Data Analysis	Identification of themes *Possible Software: Atlas Ti8*	Frequencies *Possible Software: SAS, SPSS, R*
Reporting Results	Provided in a report that presents the learned understanding of the phenomenon in narratives, photos, videos, charts, and/or graphs, etc.	Provided in a report that presents the demographics and other variables in quantitative, statistical ways (descriptive and inferential statistics, correlations, t-tests, ANOVA, regression, etc.)

ANOVA, analysis of variance; IRB, institutional review board; PTA, Parent-Teacher Association; TBI, traumatic brain injury.

REPORTING QUALITATIVE RESEARCH RESULTS

When conducted well, qualitative research provides information that is valid and reliable. Valid results in qualitative research means that those findings being presented are accurately representing the event or phenomenon of the study. Reliability in qualitative research is the same as reliability in quantitative research, which represents the reproducibility of the findings when the study is conducted again by another researcher under the same circumstances (Wolcott, 2009). Assuring the removal of bias through bracketing, identifying contradictory evidence, and triangulating data (using at least two methods to look at the same phenomenon) increases the validity of the findings. The results are required to present the evidence uncovered during the study, evidence that supports the claims that are being made by the researcher. Credibility is examined as well, providing the evidence that demonstrates the believability of the results. Although the results section is where findings are presented, how the researcher has chosen to group specific items infuses the results with a tinge of conclusion. The overall implications of the findings, however, are discussed in the conclusion or discussion section.

Data From an Interview

The researcher can explain the method in the methodology section, then use direct quotes, either sentences or full paragraphs. If the researcher wants to include the discussion from the interview, then presenting it as a script would be appropriate:

> **Researcher:** *How did hearing the voices make you feel during the simulation?*
>
> **Volunteer 1:** *At first it was okay, but after a few seconds, I felt my heart racing (volunteer 1 puts a hand up on face, which has suddenly become flushed again).*
>
> **Researcher:** *Can you describe what you are feeling now? (Volunteer 1 nods yes, eyes blinking rapidly, holding back tears.)*
>
> **Researcher:** *How about we just take a minute to breathe and relax? Is that okay with you? (Volunteer 1 breathes a big sigh and nods yes.)*
>
> **Volunteer 1:** *Yes, I think I'd like to wait a minute; maybe it affected me more than I thought. (Volunteer 1 shows a small smile. It appears that volunteer 1 is relieved to have the minute to reflect on the experience before expressing what was felt.)*

Data From Focus Groups

This can also be reported with bullet points or in charts, listing the direct quotes under the theme or researcher prompt. It can be written up as a script as well, identifying volunteer 1, volunteer 2, volunteer 3, and so on. When providing the information from a focus group, it is helpful to show how the participant's responses often reflect the group's consensus, which is easily demonstrated in the script method.

> **Researcher:** *How did hearing the voices make you feel during the simulation?*
>
> **Volunteer 1:** *At first it was okay, but after a few seconds, I felt my heart racing (volunteer 1 puts a hand up on face, which has suddenly become flushed again).*
>
> **Volunteer 2:** *I felt the same way. I tried to ignore the voices, like I ignore my little sister, but they wouldn't go away.*
>
> **Volunteer 3:** *I only heard the one that kept saying "Leave now!"— the command one.*

Volunteer 4: Yeah, that one was scary; it must be hard for someone with psychosis who is hearing a command voice. (The group nods, agreeing with volunteer 4.)

Researcher: So what did you learn from that, as a future nurse?

Volunteer 1: If a person is having an auditory hallucination, always ask what the voices are saying. (The group nods vigorously together; many say yeah or uh-huh.)

Data From Written Reflections or Other Writings

Excerpts from writing can be grouped in themes and presented to demonstrate the kinds of statements that were provided. An example from Marshall, Bliss, Evans, and Dukhan (2018) demonstrates one way for presenting these results.

Fast Facts

Qualitative Results From Written Samples

"Empathy statements ($n = 158$) were abundant in all of the self-reflections, often combined with a reflection of deeper understanding of the underlying pathology of psychosis.

- Now that I was able to experience a little insight with this simulation, my fear and anxiety from the whole thing will help me remain calm and give people with mental disorders the empathy and respect they deserve.
- Just being in the head of a patient that hears multiple voices, for only 6 seconds, allows me to appreciate them more.
- There is always a stigma with patients like this, but putting me in this situation, being able to experience what they experience on a daily basis, allows me to better understand what goes on in their heads.
- He/she fights battles every day to conduct basic everyday tasks like talking.
- I was able to step into their shoes—it was a reminder to me that their lives are not easy and that there are many things they will have to overcome in a single day."

Source: Marshall, B., Bliss, J., Evans, B., & Dukhan, O. (2018). Fostering transformation by hearing voices: Evaluating a 6-second, low-fidelity simulation. *Journal of the American Psychiatric Nurses Association, 24*(5), 426–432. doi:10.1177/1078390317750749

REPORTING QUANTITATIVE RESEARCH RESULTS

Norris, Plonsky, Ross, and Schoonen (2015) provide excellent guidelines for the reporting of quantitative methods and results. They stress how the whole methods selection should indicate the process that the researcher engaged in to come up with the final results. It stands to reason that if the process or methodology for data collection was flawed, the reliability and validity of the results will come into question.

All information that is analyzed should be presented; the statistical data (not raw data) should be presented, as well as the percentages. The descriptive and graphical analysis should include the sample size (N) and subgroup sample size (n), providing the descriptive statistics using graphs and tables where appropriate. Results are usually presented by identifying the descriptive statistics that give the reader a sense of the sample (size and composition—demographics). Statistical tests reflecting the aim/purpose of the research that would indicate manipulation of the independent variable, impact on the dependent variable, within group or between group comparisons, or specific differences in groups should be identified. Explanation of which statistical tests were carried out (parametric or nonparametric) and the reasoning behind the choices should also be presented in the results section, if not in the methods section.

The first part of the results section is always a narrative, explaining what was found. Data findings are provided to the reader in a narrative; then the researcher can place the tables and the figures. The narrative must include an explanation of missing data points, such as, for example, if 600 surveys were distributed, and 350 were returned, but only 300 of the returned surveys were eligible for analysis because 50 included missing or incomplete data.

When you use a table or a figure, it should be able to stand on its own; the reader should understand what it means just by looking at the short caption on the table itself. For figures put the title below, and for tables put the title above. When discussing a table or figure, use grammatical present tense ("The table demonstrates…"), as opposed to past tense ("The participant were provided with…").

Reporting Trends and Changes

Explain trends and direction (e.g., if something is larger/smaller, more/less, or increased/decreased) when you compare two groups. Be clear in the vocabulary you choose, identifying each of the groups (intervention or control). State what was the same in the two groups and what was different. Be specific in describing the sample or variable of interest.

REMEMBER MIXED METHODS?

Table 14.2 describes the process of research design, data collection and analysis, and presentation of results for a mixed methods study.

Table 14.2

Mixed Methods Study: From Research Design to Results	
Design	Qualitative (interview) + quantitative (survey)
Setting	Pediatrician's office + Parent teacher organization (PTO) meeting in four elementary schools near the hill
IRB Approval	Approved prior to any data collection
Sample	Purposive sample: Parents with children who have had a TBI and
	Letter sent home to all parents of students at four elementary schools, explaining the project and requesting volunteers; one parent from pre-k, kindergarten, first, second, and third grade chosen based upon availability
	All parents with children in third grade and under at four elementary schools will be provided with a survey when arriving for the PTA meeting, with a consent form and explanation of the study attached
Method of Data Collection	Videotaped or audiotaped interviews with five parents; notes taken during interview as well
	Surveys distributed to all parents arriving at the meetings; PTA president explains the anonymous survey and reason for study and tells parents that the surveys can be deposited in boxes located at the exit of the auditorium
Data Analysis	Identification of themes, descriptive statistics, frequencies, inferential statistics: t-tests, correlations and qualitative theme identification, content analysis (deductive content analysis and inductive content analysis)
Results	Provided in a report that includes both the statistical data discovered through data collection and the qualitative information in appropriate narratives and charts
	The triangulation of the data (providing at least two methods of looking at the same event) increases the depth of understanding and provides additional support for the analysis and conclusion

IRB, institutional review board; PTA, Parent–Teacher Association; PTO: Parent–Teacher Organization; TBI, traumatic brain injury.

EVALUATING THE RESULTS SECTION

When a study is conducted, whether it is transforming care at the bed-side (TCAB), a final paper, thesis, project, dissertation, or National Institutes of Health (NIH) grant, someone is going to look at the results! Too often students skip reading the results section altogether and rush into the conclusion. All those statistics, figures, and facts can seem overwhelming. Unfortunately, if a person does not know how to evaluate the results section, it is impossible to determine if what is said in the discussion is accurate.

It is said that in order to be a good writer, a person should read a lot. In order to write up a good results section, it does not hurt to start becoming a good evaluator of results sections of others. Do not be afraid of the results section! It is your best indicator of the credibility of the discussion.

Some questions to keep in your mind as you read the results section in other studies are:

1. Is the researcher only presenting the findings, or are there sentences in there that try to introduce an explanation or discussion on the outcome? ONLY the findings should be presented.
2. Is the results section organized according to the research question/purpose? Present the data that actually speak to the research question. The research question/purpose identifies the types of data that are being evaluated. If it is mixed methods, look for the variables that are identified in both the research questions.

Quantitative Design: Result Section Evaluation

The results section in quantitative design is presented in an almost formulary manner. The Fast Facts on evaluating a results section looks at the preliminary results reported in Marshall, Roberts, Donnelly, and Rutledge (2011). Look at what the question for this research study was and identify the important variables: students, knowledge of campus policies on alcohol use, attitudes toward campus policies, and relationship between campus policies on alcohol use and alcohol consumptions and campus policies and alcohol consumption social norms. This is a complex study that examines multiple variables; however, the reporting of these results (e.g., demographics and awareness) is quite clear and understandable.

Evaluating a Results Section

Question: What are students' knowledge and attitudes toward campus alcohol policies and how do they relate to alcohol consumption and alcohol social norms?

Sample: College students—on campus and off campus.

Method: Survey

RESULTS: The majority of respondents were female (63%) and White (65%) and one-half (53%) lived on campus. Almost all (99%) of the students were full time and were under the legal drinking age of 21, with the average age of the respondents being 18 years.

Table 1. Demographic Characteristics of Respondents

Characteristic	N	%
Gender		
Female	254	63
Male	148	27
Race/Ethnicity		
White	262	65
Hispanic	54	13
Black	30	7
Asian/Pacific Islander	21	5
Other	37	10
Residence		
On-campus	211	52
Off-campus	191	48

Attitudes and Knowledge:

Table 3: Awareness and Support of Campus Rules and Regulations

Item	N	(%)
Know of and support rules	158	(39)
Know of and oppose rules	56	(14)
Know of and have no opinion regarding rules	144	(36)
Do not know of rules	46	(11)

Source: Marshall, B., Roberts, K., Donnelly, J., & Rutledge, I. (2011). College student perceptions on campus alcohol policies and consumption patterns. *Journal of Drug Education, 41*(4), 345–358. doi:10.2190/DE.41.4.a

How might the results section be organized in the imaginary Jack and Jill quantitative study? The qualitative study? How about the mixed methods? What would be the same? What would be different? What would you be looking for? What kinds of results should be reported?

1. Look for the research question to help identify what kind of data was being collected.
2. In the question and aim, what variables of interest are identified? Sample? Knowledge level? Feelings? Reflections? Outcomes?
3. Does the results section start with a narrative to let you know what or who the sample comprises? If it is quantitative, is there a description of the sample with frequencies, descriptive statistics, and/or a table or chart to clarify? If it is qualitative research, has the researcher identified the approach, named the themes and concepts that were being grouped together, and provided an explanation for the process of validating the facts (i.e., interrater reliability check)? Is there a sufficient amount of documentation by the qualitative researcher related to the collection of the data? If it is mixed methods, is this clearly identified, and are all the facts presented?

See the following Fast Facts for results section from Jack and Jill.

Fast Facts

The Continuing Case of Jack and Jill: Evaluating a Results Section

Question: What is the level of parental knowledge related to the causes of and long- and short-term effects of traumatic brain injuries (TBIs), and how do they feel about TBIs?

Sample: Parents from four public schools with children in k–3 grades

Method: Survey and focus group interviews

RESULTS: The majority of respondents were female (75%) and White (65%). Almost all (95%) of the parents were in their late 30s with the average age of the respondents being 37 years old.

Table 1. Demographic Characteristics of Respondents

Characteristic	N	%
Gender		
Female	300	75
Male	100	25

(continued)

(continued)

Race/Ethnicity		
White	260	65
Hispanic	40	10
Black	40	10
Asian/Pacific Islander	20	5
Other	40	10
Schools		
School 1	100	25
School 2	100	25
School 3	100	25
School 4	100	25

Knowledge of TBI:

Table 3: Parent Knowledge of TBI by School

Item	N	(%)
Excellent knowledge of TBI	40	(10)
Some knowledge of TBI	80	(20)
Little knowledge of TBI	200	(50)
No knowledge of TBI	40	(10)

What do you think needs to be next? Why? What do you, as a reader, need to know?

ROUNDUP

The results section is a very important part of the research. It is where the findings (only the findings) are presented, without the interpretation of the researcher. It allows the reader to see what kinds of analyses were performed on the data (quantitative) and whether the presented subject matter (qualitative) was appropriate and related to the research question and study's purpose. It allows the researcher and reader to look at the data with an unbiased eye. In qualitative research the approach is examined. It should be clear if the data are chronologically or thematically presented. The results section identifies the level of the narrative and provides the evidence that any researcher bias was bracketed. The findings should also be well organized and clear to the reader. The data collected should reflect the purpose, present the demographics, and establish that the sample

205

Chapter 14   Results: What Did the Project Discover? Why Is It Important?

size was large enough for inferential statistics. Understanding the results section represents an understanding of all the pieces of the research puzzle up to now. Placing the results out for the researcher and public to see exposes the facts of the investigation. The more students or novice researchers examine the results sections of other valid and established research, the better prepared they will be to write up their own.

LINKS TO LEARN MORE

How to write the results: Part 1: https://www.youtube.com/watch?v=pKAJz3eNxbg

Normal distribution—Explained simply (part 1): https://www.youtube.com/watch?v=xgQhefFOXrM

Normal distribution—Explained simply (part 2): https://www.youtube.com/watch?v=iiRiOlkLa6A

Writing tip # 3 writing qualitative finding paragraphs: https://www.youtube.com/watch?v=mmKuvwk8x84

References

Kernler, D. (2014). *A visual representation of the Empirical (68-95-99.7) Rule based on the normal distribution* [Image file]. Retrieved from https://commons.wikimedia.org/wiki/File:Empirical_Rule.PNG

Marshall, B., Bliss, J., Evans, B., & Dukhan, O. (2018). Fostering transformation by hearing voices: Evaluating a 6-second, low-fidelity simulation. *Journal of the American Psychiatric Nurses Association, 24*(5), 426–432. doi:10.1177/1078390317750749

Marshall, B., Roberts, K., Donnelly, J., & Rutledge, I. (2011). College student perceptions on campus alcohol policies and consumption patterns. *Journal of Drug Education, 41*(4), 345–358. doi:10.2190/DE.41.4.a

Norris, J., Plonsky, L., Ross, S., & Schoonen, R. (2015). Guidelines for reporting quantitative methods and results in primary research. *Language Learning, 65*(2), 470–476. doi:10.1111/lang.12104

Wolcott, F. (2009). *Writing up qualitative research.* Thousand Oaks, CA: Sage.

15

The Conclusion of the Thesis, Project, or Dissertation: Writing the Discussion, Conclusion, and Abstract

INTRODUCTION, or *Putting the pieces of the puzzle together*

Well, welcome to the last sections of the research project: the discussion, conclusion, and abstract. The study has come a long way since identifying the Big Problem, and it is finally time to look carefully at your results to determine what they imply. The paper, report, or article that will come from this project will conclude with a discussion section and possibly also a conclusion. It is after writing up the discussion/conclusion that the researcher will compose the abstract. The abstract succinctly explains the whole project, usually in a paragraph of 100 to 500 words. Providing a discussion, reaching conclusions based upon the results of the project, and crafting the abstract is not really the end though, as you will see in Chapter 16, "The Beginning: Sharing What Was Learned With the Greater Community."

OBJECTIVES

In this chapter you will learn about:

- Writing the conclusion
- Writing the abstract

IMPORTANT DEFINITIONS

Some of the important vocabulary for this chapter includes the following:

Research Abstract: The abstract is a written summary of the research project.

Paradigm: A paradigm is a representation or example of something. It acts as a prototype or model.

Premise: A premise acts as the supporting statement toward arriving at a conclusion.

Inductive Reasoning: This kind of reasoning starts with specific observations to develop a theory. Often it is the inductive method that is used in qualitative studies (a qualitative paradigm). The inductive method reflects when a person is able to make some specific observations and then come to a generalized conclusion based upon those specific observations. In inductive reasoning, the conclusion that has been considered might, or might not, be true. Sometimes, using inductive reasoning, the conclusion might be too general (B is a pediatric nurse, nurse B likes dogs better than cats, so all pediatric nurses prefer dogs to cats).

Deductive Reasoning: This kind of reasoning starts with an accepted theory to confirm the inclusion of specific observations. It is usually deductive reasoning that is used in quantitative studies (a quantitative paradigm). When a general principle is demonstrated to be true, then specific observations that concur with the general principle will also be true. Deductive reasoning is also referred to as top-down reasoning, since what is known to be true supports the fact that the observations fall within those true principles.

WHERE DOES THE DISCUSSION/CONCLUSION FIT INTO THE RESEARCH PROCESS?

The last and final presentation of the now familiar hourglass of a research project answers this question (Figure 15.1).

THE DISCUSSION/CONCLUSION

Perhaps, at this point, some of you reading this book might have noticed that there was a little repetition connecting the chapters

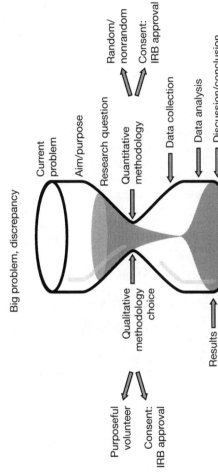

Figure 15.1 Hourglass of inquiry: The discussion and conclusion.

IRB, institutional review board.

to each other. That repetition is a trademark in writing up the discussion, which is sometimes called just a conclusion or even called the summary of your study. The reader might have forgotten, since the introduction of your topic, BIG PROBLEM, discrepancy, and research question, what the study is all about. So, the opening of your discussion/conclusion section should remind them of these things. By restating these important pieces of the study jigsaw puzzle, you lead the reader to the only piece still missing, the discussion/conclusion where you interpret the findings and describe the importance of them. A helpful hint, when writing this section, is to go back to the beginning, to the following two important questions:

- How do I know what to believe?
- How can I trust what I know?

A discussion/conclusion should be believable and trustworthy, regardless of the research methodology that was used. The discussion/conclusion should provide a decision or judgment reached through a course of scientific reasoning, which either supports or refutes the original hypothesis. The discussion/conclusion should be coherent, valid, verifiable, and credible. It should provide a review of the problem, restatement of the hypothesis, aim and research question, summary of the methodology as well as the results, and introduce the takeaways. It should also indicate limitations of the study. Finally, it should conclude with some thoughts on where the next study, on this or a related topic, should logically go.

Establishing Believability and Trustworthiness

The discussion/conclusion can only be as valid and trustworthy as the evidence it is based upon. A way to determine if you have built a study that can withstand the scrutiny of other researchers and consumers of research will be to answer the questions in Table 15.1 related to your project.

A carefully constructed study will answer these questions with a resounding YES!

Research is a process, like building a house; in order for the final result to be something that is trustworthy, all the pieces must fit together. Sometimes they do, and sometimes they do not. Despite being able to answer yes to all the questions, the researcher might learn that the evidence does not support the hypothesis. This is not a terrible thing, as long as the researcher is honest in the reporting of the evidence and provides a conclusion that explains the outcomes based in what was collected. It is often a good thing when the project results are not what are expected and demand that we

Table 15.1

Believability and Trustworthiness Questions		
Questions to ask to establish believability and trustworthiness of the conclusion	Y	N
Was the *Big Problem* and current problem identified and examined in the background?	Y	N
Was the *hypothesis* that was held at the start of the project presented?	Y	N
Did the hypothesis relate directly to the BIG PROBLEM as well as the problem at hand?	Y	N
Did the *aim* of the study reflect the *need to know* **a**spect of the discrepancy?	Y	N
When examining the *research question*, was it encapsulating the purpose of the study?	Y	N
Did the research question indicate the *variables of interest* as well as the population?	Y	N
Was the *method* chosen clear and appropriate to collect the data required?	Y	N
Was the analysis appropriate for the data collected?	Y	N
Were the results reported free of bias?	Y	N

turn toward a new direction of inquiry. Engaging in research is actively engaging in learning, discovery, and curiosity. The discussion/conclusion must reflect the integrity of the research and the researcher.

Approaches: Inductive or Deductive?

Reasoning is using logic to answer a question. Research is an exciting voyage into the world of reasoning. It directs our thinking toward defining a problem, identifying the discrepancy, and clarifying what we actually see as the current problem. If we are engaging in quantitative research, the methodology directs us toward hypothesizing, or predicting, what we think is either the cause or a way to ameliorate the problem. When we choose a qualitative approach, we seek to examine the problem or phenomenon closely and develop a theory or generalization from the evidence collected. These two methods of research usually use two distinctly different logical approaches: inductive reasoning and deductive reasoning (see Table 15.2). Knowing which approach you have

Table 15.2

Deductive and Inductive Reasoning Terminology	
Deductive Reasoning	**Inductive Reasoning**
Conclusion *must* logically follow the basic ideas or premises.	Conclusion *probably* follows from the basic premises.
When the premise statements are true, then the conclusion we expect should follow. If it does, then the theory is considered valid. If it does not, then the theory may not be a valid one.	*When the premises are true,* then the expected conclusion will probably follow. If it does, then the theory is considered strong. If it does not, then it is considered weak.
When the premises are valid and the conclusions are arrived at, the theory is considered both valid and sound. A theory based upon a valid premise, which does not yield the expected conclusion, is considered unsound.	*When the strength of the premise is considered sound,* the outcome results can be either convincing/cogent, arriving at the expected result or unconvincing/uncogent, not arriving at the expected result
When the premises are false, or invalid, the theory is considered unsound.	*If, on the other hand, the premises are found to be weak,* the theory is unconvincing/uncogent.

Source: Data from Hurley, P., & Watson, L. (2018). *A concise introduction to logic* (13th ed.). Boston, MA: Cengage Learning.

employed is an important factor when writing up the conclusion. Quantitative researchers will be starting out with a theory, setting a hypothesis forward, making observations, collecting data, analyzing the data, and confirming or refuting the hypothesis. Qualitative researchers will be starting out with the observations, establishing patterns, and then developing a possible hypothesis, which in turn will allow for theory development.

Writing Up the Discussion and/or Conclusion of the Study

It is not unusual for a student to ask how long the conclusion/discussion of a study should be. The answer is *It depends*.

If you have embarked on this project out of your own curiosity and would like to share the results in a report, the discussion/conclusion of the report should only be a paragraph or two. If, on the other hand, you are researching the topic as part of an academic requirement, the best idea is to work with your professor or project leader or dissertation chair. Different institutions have different requirements. If the report is for a grant, follow the instructions from the granting institution as they too have specific requirements for reporting findings and discussing conclusions.

Another common question is whether there needs to be a discussion and a conclusion or if one would be sufficient. Again the answer is *It depends*. It is always best to refer to the entity that the report will be going to. Some schools require one or the other sections, while other schools require both. Different journals have different formats for publication, so depending on where you might want to publish the study, the requirements will be specific to that journal. In all conditions, however, the study was done for a purpose, and part of that purpose is to share what is learned with others. Writing the discussion/conclusion can be challenging as it requires academic writing that sparingly uses words that reflect clarity of meaning.

Regardless of the amount of words that will be utilized in writing up the last section of the research report, or whether this section is under one subtitle or two, there are a couple of things that should always be included:

- Brief review of the study: aim/purpose, goal, or hypothesis
- Interpretation of the findings reported in the result section
- Any limitations encountered during the research project
- A concluding summarization from the findings
- Any practice applications or contributions to the field (nursing, healthcare, business, etc.)
- What kind of future research is indicated based upon the conclusions of this study

It is in the discussion/conclusion that the researcher has an opportunity to synthesize all that was done during the research project and provide a judgment based on the results. Getting expertise in writing up the final argument of the project, using an academic voice, can be attained by reading and critically appraising the discussion/conclusions of other studies.

Appraising Discussion/Conclusions

Closely examining the findings of other studies and purposely looking only at the discussion/conclusion sections for now can help the novice researcher begin the final construction of the report. The discussion/conclusion will include a combination of the major factors of the study, highlighting them in a clear and easily comprehendible way. This is why so many students who have not gotten a clear understanding of result interpretation and analysis often skip to the discussion and conclusion. It is this part of the report, discussion/conclusion, that translates the statistics and more complicated constructs into plain English. Despite being the place where the researcher can present the last and most convincing dialogue on the study, it is important to keep in mind that the credibility of the research is not in the final presentation. Establishing credibility in a research project begins with the choice of design and ends with the appropriate analysis of the data. The discussion/conclusion should be the summation of the argument, convincing the reader as to its veracity and importance.

Take a look at the following two appraisals in the following Fast Facts boxes: One of a qualitative research article and the other of a quantitative article. The discussion/conclusion is examined line by line for including the items needed to create a good ending argument.

Fast Facts

Appraising the Discussion and Conclusion From a Qualitative Article:

Marshall, Bliss, Evans, and Dukhan (2018): Fostering transformation by hearing voices: Evaluating a 6-second, low-fidelity simulation. *Journal of the American Psychiatric Nurses Association, 24*(5). doi:10.1177/1078390317750749

(To view this article, go to www.springerpub.com/ffresearch.)

Discussion:

Sentences 1–4: Goal stated, sample identified, brief procedural provisions given

Sentences 5–9: Limitations

Sentence 10: Review of background evidence, addition of result interpretation, and indications for future studies

Conclusion:

Sentences 11-Presentation of a theory developed, related to 6-second methodology, in changing attitudes and beliefs that in turn can change behaviors

Acknowledgments, author roles, declaration of conflict of interest, and disclosure of funding followed, preceding the references.

Fast Facts

Appraising the Discussion From a Quantitative Article:

Marshall, Roberts, Donnelly, and Rutledge (2011): College student perceptions on campus alcohol policies and consumption patterns. *Journal of Drug Education, 41*(4).

(To view this article, go to www.springerpub.com/ffresearch.)

Discussion and Conclusion are combined:
Sentences 1–4: Results restated
Sentences 5: Interpretation of results supporting theoretical hypothesis
Sentences 6–14: Explanation and interpretation of results
Sentence 15: Identification of consistency with theoretical framework
Sentences 16–21: Limitations
Sentence 22: Restatement of aim
Sentence 23: Generalization of the results
Sentence 24–33: Application to real world, supported by theoretical constructs, with suggestions added
Sentences 34–37: Recap with future suggestions for studies

The more reports and articles the researcher reads and appraises with a critical eye, the clearer the path to writing an excellent ending to the report will be. The literature review, discussed in Chapter 4, "Why We Review the Literature," provides some guidelines to reading research reports. Whether the project employed a qualitative or quantitative methodology, reviewing the discussions/conclusions of other articles and thesis to determine if the findings are properly interpreted, the limitations are clearly identified, and a final conclusion with future directions is included is imperative. This is, after all is said and done, the answer to the research question and the confirmation that the aim/purpose was achieved.

Limitations

The discussion/conclusion discusses the limitations of the study. Limitations, in this context, refer to those aspects of the study that might be a compromising factor in the believability of the results. A number of things can be identified as research limitations (Research Methodology, n.d.):

- Sample size (small)
- Sample characteristics (homogeneity, maturation issues, etc.)

- Design problems that arose during data collection
- Measurement problems
- Complications that could have affected the internal or external validity of the results
- Formulation of the study's aims and objectives
- Dearth of previous research studies

Careful crafting the research study from the very beginning can help to minimize the limitations; however, limitations are a normal part of research. These limitations should be clearly indicated and their possible effect on the results discussed. Marshall et al. (2011) included a paragraph that states, "The limitations in this study include generalizability, causality and in-depth knowledge related to student access and knowledge of specific alcohol policies and related attitudes. These results may not generalize to a more broadly representative sample of college students" (p. 354).

When the researcher can identify those shortcomings that could possibly affect the generalizability of the results and explain the influences on the outcomes that were not able to be controlled for, it reflects the honesty of the researcher and the findings. When limitations are not identified, the reader or consumer of the study might be left to imagine how the unstated, but existing, limitations might have impacted the results as well as the final conclusions being offered.

THE ABSTRACT

The abstract is the summary of the whole project. It cannot be written until the project is completed! The abstract, like the report, must follow the rules of the entity that is requiring it. Be certain that you are aware of any restrictions in words or characters or any formatting/organization requirements. The abstract is like an "elevator speech" for your study. In a short paragraph the abstract should sell your study by increasing the reader's interest in the topic, project, and outcomes. When other researchers are reviewing the literature, it will be the abstract that will be reviewed first for relevance to their study, so the clarity of the abstract is imperative. A good abstract will also use keywords, which will make the study more discoverable for others doing an online search.

There are different types of abstracts, but for now we will focus on the descriptive and informative abstracts that are routinely expected for a research paper or article. An informative abstract presents all the aspects of the study, from aim/purpose, objectives, methods, and results. A descriptive abstract includes the aim, objectives, and methods but does not include the results. Sometimes with thesis, DNP projects, capstones, and dissertations, a descriptive abstract will be included in the proposal, before data collection, analysis, and results are done.

Fast Facts

Common Elements in Constructing an Abstract

There is no one set rule; however, most abstracts have *common elements*:

Title of the study: There might be a word count limit on the title if the abstract is being submitted for publication or a presentation.
Background: Use one sentence that explains what the study is about.
Aim/purpose/objective: Why was this study conducted?
Design: How was this study conducted?
Results: What did the data show?
Conclusion: What did the resulting data mean?
Keywords: Five to 10 words that will bring other researchers on this topic to your study.

ROUNDUP

This chapter explained the important aspects of the final areas of writing for the project: the discussion/conclusion and abstract. Each entity, whether it is a professor, academic institution, journal, or funding institution, has its own specific requirements for writing up a study report and the accompanying abstract. Although there are common elements that must be included in each of these, the specifics related to the actual writing of these components must follow the instructions of the institution the study is being conducted for. The discussion/conclusion should bring together the important aspects of the study and make final determinations about what the results meant, what limitations were present, how the findings can be applied in the real world, and what kind of studies might be the logical next step to expand the knowledge even further. The abstract, which is composed after the study is completed, is the elevator speech that will sell the study to others, increasing interest and visibility.

LINKS TO LEARN MORE

Conclusions, limitations, recommendations, and further work in Master's dissertations: https://www.youtube.com/watch?v=nxjfbcFOAYw

How to write a conclusion for a research paper: https://www.wikihow.com/Write-a-Conclusion-for-a-Research-Paper

How to write a research paper abstract: https://wordvice.com/how-to-write-a-research-paper-abstract

References

Hurley, P., & Watson, L. (2018). *A concise introduction to logic* (13th ed.). Boston, MA: Cengage Learning.

Marshall, B., Bliss, J., Evans, B., & Dukhan, O. (2018). Fostering transformation by hearing voices: Evaluating a 6-second, low-fidelity simulation. *Journal of the American Psychiatric Nurses Association, 24*(5), 426–432. doi:10.1177/1078390317750749

Marshall, B., Roberts, K., Donnelly, J., & Rutledge, I. (2011). College student perceptions on campus alcohol policies and consumption patterns. *Journal of Drug Education, 41*(4), 345–358. doi:10.2190/DE.41.4.a

Research Methodology. (n.d.). *Research limitations.* Retrieved from https://research-methodology.net/research-methods/research-limitations/

16

The Beginning: Sharing What Was Learned With the Greater Community

INTRODUCTION, or *The importance of getting the word out about what you discovered*

Contrary to popular belief, writing the thesis, capstone, project, or dissertation is not the end of the research story; it is just the beginning! Your project ended with identifying what still needs to be investigated. You have done a great job, and now the gauntlet has been thrown down and the challenge presented. The bottom line is that until the word goes out about what was done, what was found, and how it will affect behaviors, attitudes, and/or knowledge moving forward, the job of the researcher is not complete. The conclusions must reach beyond the academic paper and be disseminated to professionals in the field as well as the public. It is important that what has been discovered can be applied to healthcare, not only in one place but in many. Perhaps it is your study that will ignite the curiosity of someone across the globe who wants to know more about your topic. In addition to discussing why dissemination is important, especially in research that deals with the ever-changing landscape of healthcare delivery, it will also introduce the idea of rewriting the paper to get some funding to continue as a researcher extraordinaire!

OBJECTIVES

In this chapter you will learn about:

- The ABCs of getting a paper published
- Presentations at conferences: applying results to healthcare delivery
- Ideas for getting funding to support your future research

IMPORTANT DEFINITIONS

Some of the important vocabulary for this chapter includes the following:

Blind Review: The removal of any author identification from an abstract, presentation, grant proposal, or manuscript for publication when it is to be reviewed by others in the field who are experts

Peer Review: When an abstract, presentation, grant proposal, or manuscript is evaluated by a person who is considered a peer within a specific area of specialization

DISSEMINATION (SPREADING THE NEWS)

Publishing in Articles, Books, Chapters, and Blogs: The Written Word

Many textbooks will suggest that the plan for dissemination should start alongside the identification of the project. Most of the time, just starting a research project is daunting enough, so the added stress of having to actually publish might turn some novice researchers away. Once the project is completed and the many hours that were spent to write up the different sections are behind the researcher, it is a good time to consider that maybe there is still one more thing to do.

Publish. Why not? All the hard work is done already. Go for it!

WHERE THE RESULTS FIT INTO THE RESEARCH PROCESS

This is the last and final presentation of the now familiar hourglass of a research project (Figure 16.1).

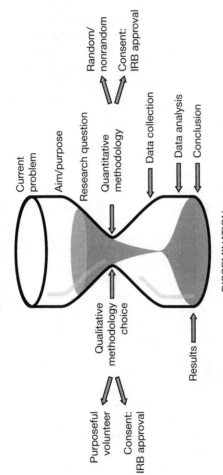

Figure 16.1 The complete hourglass of inquiry: From BIG PROBLEM to dissemination.

IRB, institutional review board.

Audience

The first task is to determine who the audience is going to be. Will this article manuscript be going to a journal that specializes in the area of your research, one that has a more general professional audience, or a magazine or newspaper? Each of these audiences will require specific language to make the study appeal to them. A good tip for finding a journal for your article would be to look at the journals that published the articles you evaluated in your literature review. If it has taken you over a year to complete your study, and if your literature is over 6 months old, you might want to do another recent search to see if anything has been published in your topic or field since you completed your study and which journals published them.

Just like reading other researchers' work when writing the discussion/conclusion, reading articles from the journals that you are interested in getting published in is very important. Many journals have a distinct voice that they use, which will be apparent after reading just a couple of articles. If you have done research that is very specific to a specialization, like psychiatric nursing or public health, it is best to look into journals that cater to an audience of professionals in that same field. Research teams that include multidisciplinary specialists can look at each of the different areas for publishing ideas, expanding the possibilities of publication.

Perhaps this experience has made you the expert in this field. As an expert you might want to consider publishing a chapter in a book, or maybe a book itself on the topic. Getting in touch with publishers looking for new topics for textbooks, self-help books, and general audience books can help you move in this direction. The audience for this kind of writing will depend on the book, chapter, and publisher.

If, on the other hand, you want to share your research directly with the public, you might want to write an article for a popular magazine, a newspaper, or a blog report. The vernacular, or language you will be using in these publications, will be very different than that used for academics. Although specialty trade journals catering to your profession will expect language reflective of academia, more general magazines, newspapers, and blogs will want the language to be quotidian, or everyday kind of speech. The audience will need the more clinical and statistical aspects of the research to be broken down using sentences that make the results of your study very clear and understandable.

Consider the morning news reports that tell about scientific outcomes to prolong life, decrease colon cancer, or improve relationships. Many journalists are not combing through journals or scientific studies, but rather the results of a study might have caught the eye of someone who considered it important enough to have it shared with the general public. Perhaps the journal editor reached out to reporters or posted something on social media, or the researcher wrote a piece for the local paper, and from there it was picked up by a reporter and presented on the morning news.

Scaling Down From a Report, Paper, or Dissertation to an Article

The original report or dissertation will usually be long, especially if it is an academic endeavor. Journals, on the other hand, will want the manuscript for articles to be manageable and publishable. Most journals will list the kinds of articles they print, the length (by words and characters) that are expected, the key sections that will be required, and the assurances that will need to be made to them regarding the originality of the work.

The Submission Process

After you choose the journal you would like to submit your manuscript to, go online and look at their Information for Authors page. Most pages will explain a little about the journal, state why you should publish with them (citing their circulation numbers), and provide other general information about their publication process, for example, peer review, standards for publication, instructions and guidelines, and possibly any publication fees (open access publications). Carefully review the submission process and read some of the other articles published by that journal to establish authenticity of publication. Chapter 4, "Why We Review the Literature," discussed the increasing number of fake and unethical publishers (FUPs). It is the author's responsibility to check whether the journal in question has been listed as a predatory journal, or if the manuscripts that are published by that journal are filled with citation errors and incorrect information. A good researcher will not want to be associated with or be published by an FUP.

Fast Facts

Considerations When Publishing With a Nursing Journal

After reading multiple articles for a research project, Nurse N decided that the *American Journal of Nursing* (*AJN*) would be a good place to publish the manuscript. Nurse N then embarked on the following pathway:

1. Goes onto the *AJN* website and reviews *AJN* author submissions

(continued)

(*continued*)

2. Checks out the information to authors page (journals.lww .com/ajnonline/Pages/informationforauthors.aspx)

3. Reads the information listed and clicked on submit a manuscript

4. Arrives at the Editorial Manager for the *AJN* page, which has files, resources, author forms, explanation about "QUERIES," author guidelines, information for first-time users, and information for people who want to become peer reviewers. There is even an "Author Tutorial" available.

5. Nurse N is a first-time user, and clicks on Register, which allows the Editorial Manager to assign a user ID and password to Nurse N for future use. After this first time, Nurse N will be a repeat user/author and will be able to log in from any computer anywhere to upload manuscripts, track the manuscript, get peer reviews, resubmit manuscripts with editorial suggestions, and receive notification of publication.

6. After careful review of the requirements, Nurse N submits a manuscript and waits to hear back from the reviewers.

Review and Resubmit: Do not be discouraged if you get a determination of "review and resubmit." It is highly unusual for a manuscript to be fully accepted on the first try. Despite the fact that the researcher has met all the conditions for the academic institution, writing for a larger group than the professor, evaluators, committee, or department demands a bit more. When the manuscript goes to peer review, it will be read by anywhere from two to five reviewers, specialists in the area of the paper's topic. Each of them will provide his or her findings in writing, usually with very clear instructions for a rewrite. The reviewers do not always agree, and it is not uncommon to get one reviewer saying excellent and important, only minor changes required, while another reviewer—concurring with the importance of the article—sends three pages of required changes.

Even the most seasoned professors with hundreds of articles meets up with what is considered the three types of peer reviewers: The first one reads the manuscript and carefully identifies where the strengths are and where the weaknesses need to be corrected. The second reviewer is too busy to provide a good review with comments the author can work on, and provides a review that is short, very general, and not that helpful in the rewrite. The third type of reviewer is considered the least helpful because it feels as though the person is placing him- or herself in a position of grandiose power over the author, either negatively writing the manuscript off with a single sentence of disapproval or going word for word through the author's writing and commenting on each sentence (Duncan, 2018).

Response to Peer Reviewers: When you are asked to resubmit, you are also asked to identify in a letter to the editor (which will be shared with the peer reviewers) what changes were made in response to the requests from the reviewers. The revised manuscript is then sent back, hopefully, to the same reviewers, who have another chance to review it. You might get the manuscript back two or three times. This process can help your writing, especially if you get constructive reviewers who nurture while helping you to rewrite. The feedback, even when it feels too stern, helps to identify where in the manuscript the writing was not clear. Keep rewriting and resubmitting until the article finds its way into print.

CONFERENCE PROCEEDINGS

Conferences are another wonderful way to disseminate the results of your project. There are two methods that conferences usually use to accept presenters: podium presentation and poster presentation. Unlike publication of the study, which requires the manuscript in its entirety for consideration, both podium and poster require only the submission of an abstract. In fact, when googling to present at a conference of your choice, put the topic or specialty area, conference, and abstract submission in the finder:

- Sigma Theta Tau conference abstract submission: www. sigmanursing.org/connect-engage/meetings-events/ calls-for-abstracts
- American Psychiatric Nurses Association conference abstract submission: www.apna.org/i4a/pages/index.cfm ?pageid=3306
- National League for Nursing (NLN) conference 2019 call for abstracts: www.nln.org/calendar/event-details/2018/12/12/ default-calendar/call-for-abstracts-2019-nln-education-summit

The website (in this case the NLN call for abstracts) will explain *the theme* of the conference (e.g., "NLN North Star: Purpose, Power and Passion"), identify *categories* ("teaching excellence, active learning...simulation"), tell what *must be in the abstract* ("All abstracts must reflect the League's core values"), state the kinds of *audiences* ("Under each topic, abstracts should be geared to one of two audiences: emerging educators and more seasoned educators"), and *state the deadline* for submission (December 12, 2019, 11:59 p.m.).

Each conference will have its own set of rules, but using the abstract already crafted for the paper, it is not difficult to reword it to fit the requirements of the conference proceedings.

Poster

If the submission is for a poster, the project's background, methods, results, and discussion are formatted to a poster template (see Figure 16.2). The researcher is expected to make the poster (many universities will print the poster for faculty and students) and bring it to the conference. Some conferences, like the DNP conference, accept and present their posters in digital form. Both types require that the author stand by the poster for a duration of time and speak to people who are circulating in the poster area. It is usually a one-to-one group, so if the author is worried about a public presentation, this way is not intimidating at all.

Presentation

The same abstract that you would submit for a poster is what is also submitted for a presentation. Usually the presentation might involve one to five or more presenters on a specific topic. If the abstract is accepted as a sole presenter, the presentation might be anywhere from 45 minutes to 1.5 hours. If the presentation is part of a group or panel, the amount of time will vary, typically between 15 and 20 minutes. The size of the audience will depend on the size of the conference and the interest that is generated by your title, abstract, and topic. Remember, the abstract is the elevator speech that will sell the idea to the possible audience members. The presentation might have as few as five attendees and as many as a couple of hundred; in any case the presenter must be prepared to deliver an excellent speech that explains the study and respects the delivery time frame.

Application to Healthcare

Application to healthcare is only discussed in the discussion/conclusion of the research paper; however, once you have entered the presentation arena, the application of the research findings become the focus of the audience: what was discovered and how can it be used to improve practice, healthcare, patient's recovery, education, and so on. Pace your presentation, whether poster or presentation, to give enough time to talk about the application of your findings and allow the audience to ask questions. Frequently it is when an author prepares a presentation that the importance of the findings to the delivery of care becomes more apparent. It is also not unusual for the

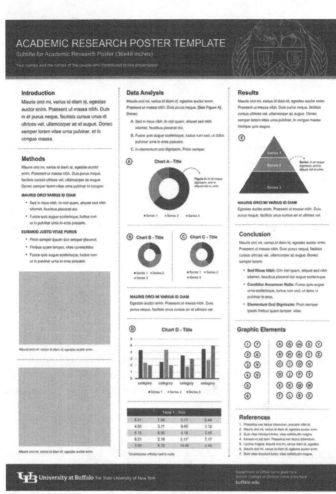

Figure 16.2 Example of an academic poster template.

Source: University at Buffalo. (n.d.). *Research poster template*. Retrieved from http://www.buffalo.edu/brand/resources-tools/ub-templates-and-tools/research-poster.html

audience to provide some great ideas about where the next research project is hiding!

GRANT FUNDING

Research is the foundation of knowledge and as such demands to be engaged in and funded. Funding comes from a variety of different sources, from the small grants that are provided by individuals and schools, to the larger grants that come from the state and federal government. There are many funding organizations, most of which seek to fund research by a researcher who has conducted valid, reliable, trustworthy research in an area of the funders' interest (see Table 16.1).

You have now entered the arena of a researcher who has conducted, written up, and presented the findings of original research. It is your responsibility to find the funders; they will not be coming to find you. It is always good to have a plan in research, and finding funding is no exception. The pathways include looking at general funding programs for nurses,

Specialists should check their associations for funding opportunities and be open about seeking funding when presenting the research to a group of people. There just might be someone in that crowd who has the connections needed to get the funding to continue the research.

GRANT WRITING

Once funding sources have been identified, it is wise to start considering how to turn your research paper into an excellent grant. Grant writing is a field of writing in itself, and many institutions have hired specialists in grant writing to secure the desired funding for a project. It is common for those consultants to be available to healthcare staff, students, and faculty through the institution's office of sponsored projects. Your success in finding funding is their success as well.

If you do not have the good fortune to have a grant writer on your team, the best bet for getting your first funding is to apply for a small grant from a funding agency specific to your project. For example, a psychiatric nurse seeking funding might look to the American Psychiatric Nurses Association (APNA; www.apna.org/i4a/pages/index.cfm?pageid=3532) or the International Society of Psychiatric Nurses (ISPN; www.ispn-psych.org/scholarships-grants). Nurse practitioners might seek funding from the American Association of Nurse Practitioners (AANP; www.aanp.org/education/professional-funding-support). These small grants allow the novice researcher to write a grant proposal, following the instructions and guidelines carefully, get feedback from the reviewers (yes, there is a blind review of the abstracts and the proposals), and get funded for the first time. In some instances, the fact that you have not yet been funded will place you in a preferred pile of applications.

Table 16.1

General Funding Opportunities for Nursing and Healthcare Providers

Funder	Research Funding	Amount	Links
NLN	NLN Nursing Education: Mary Ann Rizzolo Doctoral Research Award	Up to $30,000 $2.500 $5,000	www.nln.org/professional-development-programs/grants-and-scholarships/nursing-education-research-grants/nln-nursing-education-research-grants-proposal-guidelines
	Multiple small grants (10)		www.nln.org/professional-development-programs/grants-and-scholarships/nursing-education-research-grants/dr-mary-anne-rizzolo-nln-doctoral-dissertation-dnp-project-award
			www.sigmanursing.org/advance-elevate/research/research-grants/sigma-grants
Sigma Theta Tau	Multiple grants	Different amounts	www.sigmanursing.org/advance-elevate/research/research-grants
ANA	Multiple grants	Different amounts	www.nursingworld.org/foundation/programs/nursing-research-grants/
Physician assistants	Multiple grants from different organizations	Different amounts	paeaonline.org/advocacy/funding-opportunities/
Public health funding resources	Multiple grants	Different amounts	www.aspph.org/teach-research/funding-opportunities/
Non-NIH funding for students, faculty, and travel	Multiple grants	Different amounts	www.fic.nih.gov/Funding/NonNIH/Pages/health-professionals.aspx

ANA, American Nurses Association; NIH, National Institutes of Health; NLN, National League for Nursing.

Helpful Tips on Writing Your First Grant Proposal

1. Have a plan: Know who you are seeking funds from and what exactly they have funded before.

2. Find a mentor: Anything is complicated the first time around, and finding someone who can help you to navigate the process is ideal. Volunteer to work on a grant that is being written by someone who has been getting funding.

3. Network at conferences: Find people who are interested in your topic, get their professional cards, and pick their brains about where funding might be available. Meet with them if possible, and get them to be your mentor.

4. Utilize professional organizations: Look into organizations where you are already a member, and join organizations that have a mission that is similar to your interests and specialties. Many professional organizations have grant writing programs online and conferences specifically geared to new researchers seeking funding.

5. Become a grant reviewer: Look at the kinds of grants that you feel might be right for you in the future, and volunteer to be a grant reviewer so that you can become an expert in understanding what is expected in the proposal.

6. Collaborate with others: Share the information and the responsibilities of writing the grant. Make sure that the end result speaks with one voice.

7. FOLLOW DIRECTIONS! Grant applications are very specific from the font and size of the letters to the number of pages and words that will be accepted. Focus on the project, not on yourself, and keep your wordsmithing radar on. Provide the facts, just the facts, and make sure that the flow of the project—from BIG PROBLEM to Conclusion—is coherent.

8. Keep trying: Do not let a rejection stop you. Perseverance pays off; after all you finished the project, didn't you?

ROUNDUP

Welcome to the beginning of your research life where a little curiosity can end up as a National Institutes of Health funded project! Getting the information from your study out to the public is how the care and treatment of patients and consumers has been able to grow and flourish. Dissemination of information is the foundation of progress and innovation. This chapter presented some of the many avenues that will be opening up to you as you embrace research and become part of the profession committed to improving care through evidence-based practices in a world where the science is evolving and the frontier of healthcare is changing every day. Welcome to this brave new world of research!

LINKS TO LEARN MORE

Giving an effective poster presentation: https://www.youtube.com/watch?v=vMSaFUrk-FA

How to write a research grant proposal step by step: https://www.youtube.com/watch?v=9g9CyCENZso

7 PowerPoint tips and conference PPT samples & examples: https://www.youtube.com/watch?v=sL4EEmYqYKg

Reference

Duncan, M. (2018). Advice: The 3 types of peer reviewers. *The Chronicle of Higher Education.* Retrieved from https://www.chronicle.com/article/The-3-Types-of-Peer-Reviewers/243698

University at Buffalo. (n.d.). *Research poster template.* Retrieved from http://www.buffalo.edu/brand/resources-tools/ub-templates-and-tools/research-poster.html

Index

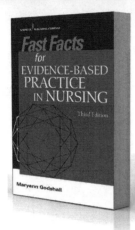
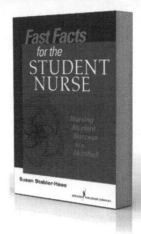
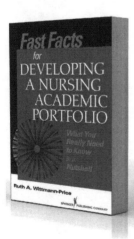
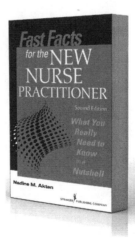